FAST METABOLISM DIET

BURN THE BASS!

Turboboost Your Metabolism and Fortify Your Immune System with Proven Meal Plans, Recipes, and Intermittent Fasting For Amazing Results

ADAN FORD

Table of Contents

PART I 12

WHAT IS METABOLISM? 13

PHASE 1 16

BREAKFAST 16

CINNAMON APPLE QUINOA 16

LUNCH 17

MASHED CHICKPEA SALAD 17

DINNER 18

SLOW COOKER SPAGHETTI AND MEATBALLS 18

PHASE 2 21

BREAKFAST 22

KOREAN ROLLED OMELETTE 22

LUNCH 22

MARINATED TOFU WITH PEPPERS AND ONIONS 22

DINNER 24

ROAST BEEF AND VEGETABLES 24

PHASE 3 25

BREAKFAST 25

BERRY COBBLER WITH QUINOA 25

LUNCH 26

ITALIAN TUNA SALAD 26

DINNER 27

SHEET PAN STEAK AND VEGGIES 27

DOS AND DON'TS 28

PART II 32

Chapter 1: Meal Planning 101 33

Make a Menu 34

Plan around Ads 34

Go Meatless Once Per Week 34

Use Ingredients That You Already Have On Hand 35

Avoid Recipes that Call for a Special Ingredient 35

Use Seasonal Foods 35

Make Use of Leftovers and Extra Portions 36

Eat What You Enjoy 36

Chapter 2: 1 Month Meal Plan 37

Week 1: Success is no accident—you have to reach for it 37

Mediterranean Breakfast Sandwich 37

Greek Chicken Bowls 39

Ratatouille 41

Snack Platter 43

Week 2: Self-belief and effort will take you to what you want to achieve 46

Breakfast Quesadilla 46

Greek Orzo Salad 47

One Pot Mediterranean Chicken 49

Mediterranean Nachos 51

Week 3: The harder you work, the greater the success 52

Breakfast Tostadas 52

Roasted Vegetable Bowl 53

Mediterranean Chicken 55

Baked Phyllo Chips.. 57

Week 4: You don't need perfection—you need effort.................... 57

Mini Omelets 58

Basil Shrimp Salad.. 60

Mediterranean Flounder.. 61

Nutty Energy Bites 62

Week 5: Transformation Happens One Day at a Time 64

Mediterranean Breakfast Bowl.. 64

Chicken Shawarma Pita Pockets 66

Turkey Mediterranean Casserole.. 67

Heirloom Tomato and Cucumber Toast.. 68

Chapter 3: Maintaining Your Diet..**69**

Find Your Motivation.. 70

Remind Yourself Why You are Eating Healthily 70

Eat Slowly.. 71

Keep Yourself Accountable 71

Remember Your Moderation.. 72

Identify the Difference between Hunger and Craving 72

Stick to the Meal Plan.. 73

Drink Plenty of Water 74

Eat Several Times Per Day 74

Fill Up on Protein.. 75

Keep Only Healthy Foods.. 75

Eat Breakfast Daily 76

PART III..**77**

Chapter 1: Muscle Mass 78

1.1. How Muscle is Built 79

Chapter 2: The Upper Body 80

2.1 The Classic Push-Up 80

2.2 Chair-Dips 81

2.3 Diamond Push-Ups 82

Chapter 3: The Core 82

3.1 Plank 84

3.2 Reverse Crunch 85

3.3 Mountain Climber 86

Chapter 4: The Lower Body 87

4.1 The Lunge 88

4.2 Squat 89

4.3 The Bridge 90

Chapter 5: Putting it all Together 91

Monday Morning Before Work: 92

Monday Lunch: 93

Monday Evening: 93

Chapter 6: On Your Diet 95

PART IV 98

CHAPTER ONE 99

CHAPTER TWO 103

A Loop 104

Problems 105

CHAPTER THREE 107

Eating Habits 107

Smoking Habits 109

Drinking Habits 110

Using your Triggers 111

CHAPTER FOUR 113

A Big Break 115

Classical Conditioning 120

Procrastination 121

Be Prepared 123

CHAPTER FIVE 124

CHAPTER SIX 132

The Three R's 133

Step by Step 135

Switch Bad for Good 137

CHAPTER SEVEN 140

CHAPTER EIGHT 144

Use it or lose it 145

CHAPTER NINE 154

Simple meditation practice 158

PART V 162

Chapter 1: Identifying the Mediterranean Diet 163

Defining the Mediterranean Lifestyle 164

The Rules of the Mediterranean Diet 165

Chapter 2: Savory Mediterranean Meals 168

Mediterranean Feta Mac and Cheese 168

Chickpea Stew 168

Savory Mediterranean Breakfast Muffins 169

Mediterranean Breakfast Bake 170

Mediterranean Pastry Pinwheels 171

Chapter 3: Sweet Treats on the Mediterranean Diet 172

Greek Yogurt Parfait 172

Overnight Oats 173

Apple Whipped Yogurt 174

Chapter 4: Gourmet Meals on the Mediterranean Diet 175

Garlic-Roasted Salmon and Brussels Sprouts 175

Walnut Crusted Salmon with Rosemary 176

Spaghetti and Clams 177

Braised Lamb and Fennel 178

Mediterranean Cod 180

Baked Feta with Olive Tapenade 181

Chapter 5: 30-Minutes or Less Meals 182

Vegetarian Toss Together Mediterranean Pasta Salad 182

Vegetarian Aglio e Olio and Broccoli 183

Cilantro and Garlic Baked Salmon 184

Harissa Pasta 185

1 Hour Baked Cod 186

Grilled Chicken Mediterranean Salad 187

Lemon Herb Chicken and Potatoes One Pot Meal 189

Vegetarian Mediterranean Quiche 191

Herbed Lamb and Veggies 192

Chicken and Couscous Mediterranean Wraps 193
Sheet Pan Shrimp 195
Mediterranean Mahi Mahi 197
Chapter 7: Slow Cooker Meals 198
Slow Cooker Mediterranean Chicken 198
Slow Cooker Vegetarian Mediterranean Stew 200
Vegetarian Slow Cooker Quinoa.. 202
Slow-Cooked Chicken and Chickpea Soup 204
Slow Cooked Brisket.. 206
Vegan Bean Soup with Spinach 207
Moroccan Lentil Soup 208
Chapter 8: Vegetarian and Vegan Meals 210
Vegetarian Greek Stuffed Mushrooms 210
Vegetarian Cheesy Artichoke and Spinach Stuffed Squash............. 211
Vegan Mediterranean Buddha Bowl... 213
Vegan Mediterranean Pasta 215
Vegetarian Zucchini Lasagna Rolls 217
Vegetarian Breakfast Sandwich.. 218
Vegan Breakfast Toast 220
Vegetarian Shakshouka 221

PART I

WHAT IS METABOLISM?

Metabolism is typically used when we are describing different chemical reactions that help to maintain healthy organisms and cells. There are two types of metabolism:

- Anabolism: the synthesis of the compounds that the cell need.
- Catabolism: the breaking down of the molecules to get energy.

Metabolism is closely linked to a person's nutrition and how they use their available nutrients. Bioenergetics tells us how our metabolic or biochemical paths for our cells use energy. Forming energy is a vital component in metabolism.

Good nutrition is the key to metabolism. Metabolism requires nutrients so they can break down to produce energy. This energy is needed to make new nucleic acids, proteins, etc.

Diets need nutrients like sulfur, phosphorus, nitrogen, oxygen, hydrogen, carbon, and 20 other inorganic elements. These elements are received from proteins, lipids, and carbohydrates. Water, minerals, and vitamins are necessary.

Your body gets carbs in three different ways from food: sugar, cellulose, and starch. Sugars and starches form essential sources of energy for us humans.

Body tissues need glucose for everyday activities. Sugars and carbs give off glucose by metabolism or digestion.

Most people's diet is half carbs. These carbs typically come from macaroni, pasta, potatoes, bread, wheat, rice, etc.

The tissue builders of the body are proteins. Proteins are found in every cell of the human body. Proteins help with enzymes that carry out needed reactions, hemoglobin formation to carry the oxygen, functions, cell structure, and many other functions within the body. Proteins are needed to supply nitrogen for DNA, producing energy, and RNA genetic material.

Protein is necessary for nutrition since they have amino acids. The human body can't synthesize eight of these, and they are amino acids that are essential to us.

These amino acids are:

- Threonine
- Valine
- Phenylalanine
- Isoleucine
- Leucine
- Methionine
- Tryptophan
- Lysine

Foods that have the best quality of protein are grains, vegetables, meats, soybeans, milk, and eggs.

Fats are a more condensed form of energy. They make twice the amount of energy as proteins or carbs.

These are the functions of fats:

- Provide a reserve for energy.
- Help to absorb fat soluble vitamins.
- Forms a protection insulation and cushion around vital organs.
- Helps to form a cellular structure.

The fatty acids that are required include unsaturated acids, such as arachidonic, linolenic, and linoleic acids. These are needed in the diet. Cholesterol and saturated fats have been associated with heart disease and arteriosclerosis.

Minerals found in food don't give you energy, but they do play a role in your bodies pathways and are important regulators. There are more than 50 elements that can be found in the body. Only 25 have been deemed essential so far. Deficiency in these could produce specific symptoms. These are the essential minerals:

- Iodine
- Fluorine
- Magnesium
- Zinc
- Manganese
- Cobalt
- Copper
- Chloride ions
- Potassium
- Sodium
- Iron
- Phosphorus
- Calcium

Vitamins are known as organic compounds that the human body is unable to synthesize by itself, so they need to be found within your diet. These are the most important vitamins in metabolism:

- Pantothenic Acid
- Nicotinic acid or Niacin
- B2 or riboflavin
- Vitamin A

Metabolism's chemical reactions are grouped within your metabolic pathways. This gives the chemicals that come from your nutrition to be changed through several different steps along with another chemical. This is done with a series of enzymes.

Enzymes are important for your metabolism because they give organisms the ability to achieve the reactions that they need for energy. These also work along with the others that release energy. Enzymes are basically catalysts that let these reactions happen efficiently and quickly.

PHASE 1

While on this diet you will rotate the way you eat between three phases:

- Phase One – Monday and Tuesday:
- Phase Two – Wednesday and Thursday:
- Phase Three – Friday, Saturday, and Sunday:
- Repeat this for four weeks.

Every phase focuses on different healthy, whole foods to help reduce your liver stress, calm your adrenal glands, and feed your thyroid. Now, let's look at phase one and some recipes to get you started.

Phase One – low-fat, moderate-protein, high-glycemic

One of the main things that phase one will help you with is by regulating your adrenal glands. The adrenal glands secrete stress hormones, which is only useful when you are in immediate danger. When you aren't in danger, all it will do for you is raise your cortisol level, which causes weight gain.

In phase one, you will eat higher glycemic fruits because they stimulate your pituitary gland, which is your pleasure center. This releases endorphins which will reduce anxiety and stress.

In phase one you will also need to do some cardio, this will help to reduce cortisol levels even more.

BREAKFAST

CINNAMON APPLE QUINOA

Serves: 2

Ingredients:

Honey

2 tsp cinnamon

2 large apples

1 ½ c water

½ c quinoa

Instructions:

Prepare the apples by coring and peeling. Chop the prepared apples into small pieces.

Place the apples, quinoa, and water into a pot. Allow the mixture to come to a boil. Place the lid on the pot and turn the heat down to a simmer. Let cook for 20 to 25 minutes. The apples should be soft, and the quinoa should have absorbed all the water.

Mix in the cinnamon and divide between two bowls.

Drizzle the top with some more cinnamon and honey.

LUNCH

MASHED CHICKPEA SALAD

Serves: 2

Ingredients:

Pepper and salt to your taste

1 ½ tbsp sunflower seeds

½ lemon, juiced

½ tsp garlic, minced

3 tbsp Dijon

2 tbsp cilantro

½ c kale, chopped

¼ c red onion, chopped

1/3 of an apple, chopped

2 celery stalks, chopped

15-oz chickpeas, rinsed and drained

1 carrot, shredded

Instructions:

Shred your carrot in a food processor and place in a large bowl.

Place the chickpeas in the processor and pulse a couple of times until well blended, but a little chunky. If you want, you can just use a potato masher.

Place chickpeas and the rest of the ingredients in the bowl with the carrot. Mix everything together and add pepper and salt to your taste.

DINNER

SLOW COOKER SPAGHETTI AND MEATBALLS

Serves: 6

Ingredients:

Meatballs:

½ tsp pepper

1 tsp salt

½ c breadcrumbs

2 eggs

1 ½ tsp oregano

¼ c parsley, minced

3 minced garlic

½ onion, grated

1 ½ lb lean ground beef

Sauce:

16-oz whole wheat spaghetti drained and cooked

4 basil leaves, sliced

14-oz crushed tomatoes

28-oz crushed tomatoes

½ tsp pepper

½ tsp salt

½ tsp sugar

4-oz tomato paste

1 tsp oregano

1 onion, chopped

3 minced garlic cloves

1 tbsp olive oil

Instructions:

Meatballs:

Your oven should be at 350. Spray a baking sheet with nonstick spray.

Mix the pepper, salt, breadcrumbs, eggs, oregano, parsley, garlic, onion, and beef together.

For the meat mixture into balls. Place them on the baking sheet, evenly spaced.

Bake until they are almost cooked, about 12 to 15 minutes. Transfer your meatballs to your slow cookers and scrape off bits of fat from the bottom of the meatballs.

Sauce:

Place the oil in a pan and heat. Place in the garlic and cook for a few seconds.

Mix in the oregano and onion. Cooking for about three minutes, the onions should be soft.

Stir in the pepper, salt, sugar, and tomato paste and cook another two minutes.

Mix in the basil and crushed tomatoes. Pour the mixture over the meatballs in your cooker.

Cook for five hours at low. Serve the mixture over your cooked spaghetti.

PHASE 2

Phase 2 – low-fat, low-carb, high-veggie, high-protein

Lean proteins provide the ingredients that create amino acids within the body. Alkaline vegetables provide enzymes and phytonutrients that break down the proteins. The amino acids are converted into muscle.

Muscles are insatiable. They need lots of fuel. The more muscle you have, the more fat you are going to burn. Muscle works for you. It burns fat that has been stored as fuel to help melt away stubborn fat. More muscle means higher metabolic rate. Muscle-building is about weight training. You can use your body weight, hand weight, weight machines, or dumbbells.

When you eat lean proteins such as chicken, fish, turkey, bison, and beef, the stomach will start to secrete pepsinogen that converts into the enzyme pepsin. This pepsin will start breaking down the protein into amino acids.

This phase isn't all about eating protein. If you were to eat nothing but protein, your body's pH balance would begin to be far too acidic and you will start to feel ill. To balance out this protein, you will be eating a lot of alkalizing vegetables like collard greens, cucumbers, spinach, kale, broccoli, and cabbage. These vegetables give the body more alkaline thus bringing the body's pH into balance.

The other good things happening in this phase is all the vitamin C that you are consuming is strengthening the adrenal glands, and we know that strong adrenal glands react less to stress.

Iodine and taurine in the vegetables will nourish the thyroid thus prepping it to release the fat-burning hormones that will be coming in the next phase.

BREAKFAST

KOREAN ROLLED OMELETTE

Serves: 1

Ingredients:

Roasted seaweed

2 pinches salt

3 eggs

½ tsp butter

Instructions:

Whisk the eggs together with some salt.

Butter a pan lightly.

Heat the pan and pour in the whisked eggs.

Let them cook until they are almost set, then place a sheet of seaweed on top.

Take a spatula and lift an edge of the egg over the seaweed. Continue to roll the egg over the seaweed. Allow it to cool slightly and then slice into one-inch pieces.

LUNCH

MARINATED TOFU WITH PEPPERS AND ONIONS

Serves: 4

Ingredients:

3 red bell peppers, seeded and sliced

1 red onion, sliced into ¼-inch thick rounds

1 tbsp honey

4 tbsp EVOO, divided

1 lb block medium tofu, sliced into ½-inch slices

Pepper and salt

¾ tsp paprika, divided

3 ½ tsp cumin, divided

¼ c garlic, minced

2/3 c lime juice

¾ c cilantro, chopped

Instructions:

Your oven should be at 450. Place foil onto a baking sheet. Mix ½ teaspoon paprika, 3 teaspoon cumin, garlic, lime juice, and ¼ cup cilantro together. Sprinkle with pepper and salt. Pour half of the marinade into a baggie. Place in the tofu. Seal the bag and shake so everything is coated. Allow to marinate at room temp for ten to fifteen minutes, flip over occasionally.

While that marinates, place the rest of the marinade in your blender. Add in honey, two tablespoons oil, and ¼ cup of cilantro. Mix until smooth, and add in pepper and salt to taste.

Mix the peppers and onion together in a bowl and season with pepper, salt, ¼ teaspoon paprika, ½ teaspoon cumin, and two tablespoons of oil.

Drain the marinade off the tofu. Sprinkle both sides with pepper and salt and place on the prepared baking sheet. Add the vegetables to the baking sheet next to the tofu.

Bake for 20 to 25 minutes, stirring the veggies a couple of times until everything is tender.

Divide the tofu and veggies among plates and top with sauce and the rest of the cilantro.

DINNER

ROAST BEEF AND VEGETABLES

Serves: 6

Ingredients:

1 lb red potatoes, halved

1 bulb fennel, thinly sliced

1 red onion, sliced

Pepper

2 tsp rosemary, chopped

Salt

2 tbsp balsamic vinegar

3 tbsp EVOO

3 lb beef rump roast, trimmed of fat

Instructions:

Your oven should be at 375. Brush the beef with a tablespoon of vinegar and oil. Then season with ½ teaspoon pepper, a teaspoon of rosemary, and two teaspoons of salt. Coat the potatoes, onion, and fennel with the rest of the salt, pepper, rosemary, vinegar, and oil. Place the veggies on the bottom of a nine by thirteen inch pan. Place the roast, fat side up, on the vegetables.

Cook until a thermometer reads 125 degrees Fahrenheit, and 1 ¼ to 1 ½ hours. Place the meat on a cutting board and rest for about ten minutes. Turn your oven up to 450. Stir the veggies and let them cook for another ten minutes. Slice the beef and serve along with the vegetables.

PHASE 3

Phase 3 – low-glycemic fruit, moderate protein, moderate carb, high healthy fat

It sounds counter-intuitive, but healthy fats from raw seeds, olive oil, avocados, and raw nuts will trigger your body to burn the dietary fat and the stored fat. You have kept your fat intake low but flooded your body with nutrients from efficient proteins, alkalizing vegetables, and whole grains. You haven't been eating fats, and your body has been burning the stored fat for energy. You might have noticed that your clothes are fitting somewhat looser, but if your body catches on, and no dietary fats are coming in, it will start to store fat again instead of burning it.

Salmon helps to promote healthy hormone balance in your adrenal and thyroid glands. Other nutrients in healthy fats will start to slow gastric emptying. This helps you feel fuller longer and stimulates the pituitary glands, and hypothalamus releases feel-good hormones and allows your body to feel satisfied and full.

BREAKFAST

BERRY COBBLER WITH QUINOA

Serves: 4

Ingredients:

1 c strawberries, frozen

2 c blackberries, frozen

¼ tsp cinnamon

¼ c almond milk

¼ c maple syrup

1 tsp vanilla

¼ c ground flaxseed

½ c coconut oil

½ c chopped walnuts

½ c quinoa flour

½ c cooked quinoa

1 c dry oats

Instructions:

Your oven should be at 375.

Mix all the ingredients together, except for the berries.

Place the berries in a nine by nine baking dish and then top with the quinoa mixture.

Cook for 35 to 40 minutes or until it has browned. You can also serve with a drizzle of honey and a dollop of Greek yogurt.

LUNCH

ITALIAN TUNA SALAD

Serves: 2

Ingredients:

¼ tsp salt

1 tbsp lemon juice

1 minced garlic clove

¼ c chopped green olives

¼ c red onion, diced

½ sweet yellow pepper, diced

3-oz black olives, sliced

½ c parsley leaves, chopped

1 c diced tomatoes

2 cans Yellowfin Tuna in Olive oil, not drained

Instructions:

Place the tuna into a bowl and break up the pieces. Mix in the rest of the ingredients. You can serve on a bun or a bed of lettuce.

DINNER

SHEET PAN STEAK AND VEGGIES

Serves: 6

Ingredients:

2 lb top sirloin

Pepper and salt

1 tsp thyme

3 minced garlic cloves

2 tbsp olive oil

16-oz broccoli florets

2 lb red potatoes

Instructions:

Your oven should be set to broil. Grease a baking sheet lightly.

Parboil the potatoes for 12 to 15 minutes and drain.

Place the broccoli and potatoes on the baking sheet. Drizzle with pepper, salt, thyme, garlic, and olive oil and toss.

Sprinkle the steak with pepper and salt and place on the baking sheet between the veggies.

Broil the steak until browned, this should take about four to five minutes on each side.

DOS AND DON'TS

Avoid these foods in all phases:

- Fat-free "diet" foods – this includes zero-cal, fat-free, or diet foods
- Artificial sweeteners
- Fruit juices and dried fruit
- Alcohol
- Caffeine – if you have to have coffee, use organic decaffeinated
- Refined sugars
- Dairy
- Corn
- Non-sprouted wheat

Phase 1:

- Meals: 3 meals and 2 fruit snacks
    - Breakfast: fruit and grain, 30 minutes after waking up
    - Fruit snack
    - Lunch: vegetable, fruit, protein, and grain
    - Fruit snack
    - Dinner: vegetable, protein, and grain
- Organic when possible

- All fruits and veggies
- Protein – veggie and animal
    - Lean meat
    - Lean poultry
    - Lean fish
    - Eggs – white only
    - Beans
- Plenty or spices, herbs, broth, and condiments
- Grains
    - Sprouted and whole wheat
- Water
- No fats

Phase 2:

- Meals
    - Breakfast: veggie and protein, 30 minutes after your get up
    - Protein snack
    - Lunch: veggie and protein
    - Protein snack
    - Dinner: veggie and protein
- Low-glycemic vegetables
- Lemon and limes

- Animal protein:
    - Lean meat
    - Lean poultry
    - Lean fish
    - Shellfish
    - Eggs- white only
- No vegetable proteins
- Condiments, spices, herbs, and broth
- No starches or grains
- No fats
- Water

Phase 3:

- Meals
    - Breakfast: veggie, grain, protein, or fat 30 minutes after waking
    - Protein, fat, or veggie snack
    - Lunch: fruit, veggie, protein, or fat
    - Protein, fat, or veggie snack
    - Dinner: starch, grain, veggie, protein, or fat
- All veggies
- Low-glycemic fruits
- Animal and veggie protein

    - Any meat
    - Liver
    - Poultry
    - Fish
    - Shellfish
    - Eggs
    - Beans
    - Seeds and nuts
    - Non-dairy proteins
- Whole starches and grains
- Condiments, spices, herbs, and broth
- Healthy fats
- Water

PART II

Chapter 1: Meal Planning 101

Sticking to a diet is something that is not the easiest in the world. When it comes down to it, we struggle to change up our diets on a whim. It might be that for the first few days, you are able to stick to it and make sure that you are only eating those foods that are better for you, but over time, you will get to a point where you feel the pressure to cave in. You might realize that sticking to your diet is difficult and think that stopping for a burger on your way home won't be too bad. You might think that figuring out lunch or dinner is too much of a hassle, or you realize that the foods that you have bought forgot a key ingredient that you needed for dinner.

The good news is, you have an easy fix. When you are able to figure out what you are making for yourself for your meals well in advance, you stop having to worry so much about the foods that you eat, what you do with them, and what you are going to reach for when it's time to eat. You will be able to change up what you are doing so that you can be certain that the meals that you are enjoying are good for you, and you won't have to worry so much about the stress that goes into it. Let's take a look at what you need to do to get started with meal planning so that you can begin to do so without having to think too much about it.

Make a Menu

First, before you do anything, make sure that you make a menu! This should be something that you do on your own, or you should sit down with your family to ask them what they prefer. If you can do this, you will be able to ensure that you've got a clear-cut plan. When you have a menu a week in advance, you save yourself time and money because you know that all of your meals will use ingredients that are similar, and you won't have to spend forever thinking about what you should make at any point in time.

Plan around Ads

When you do your menu, make it a point to glance through the weekly ads as well. Typically, you will find that there are plenty of deals that you can make use of that will save you money.

Go Meatless Once Per Week

A great thing to do that is highly recommended on the Mediterranean Diet is to have a day each week where you go meatless for dinner. By doing so, you will realize that you can actually cut costs and enjoy the foods more at the same time. It is a great way to get that additional fruit and veggie content into your day, and there are plenty of healthy options that are out there for you. You just have to commit to doing so. In the meal plans that you'll see below, you will notice that there will be a meatless day on Day 2 every week.

Use Ingredients That You Already Have On Hand

Make it a point to use ingredients that you already have on hand whenever possible. Alternatively, make sure that all of the meals that you eat during the week use very similar ingredients. When you do this, you know that you're avoiding causing any waste or losing ingredients along the way, meaning that you can save money. The good news is, on the Mediterranean diet, there are plenty of delicious meals that enjoy very similar ingredients that you can eat.

Avoid Recipes that Call for a Special Ingredient

If you're trying to avoid waste, it is a good idea for you to avoid any ingredients in meals that are not going to carry over to other meals during your weekly plan. By avoiding doing so, you can usually save yourself that money for that one ingredient that would be wasted. Alternatively, if you find that you really want that dish, try seeing if you can freeze some of it for later. When you do that, you can usually ensure that your special ingredient at least didn't go to waste.

Use Seasonal Foods

Fruits and veggies are usually cheaper when you buy them in season, and even better, when you do so, you will be enjoying a basic factor of the

Mediterranean diet just by virtue of enjoying the foods when they are fresh. Fresher foods are usually tastier, and they also tend to carry more vitamins and minerals because they have not had the chance to degrade over time.

Make Use of Leftovers and Extra Portions

One of the greatest things that you can do when it comes to meal planning is to make use of your leftovers and make-ahead meals. When you do this regularly, making larger portions than you need, you can then use the extras as lunches and dinners all week long, meaning that you won't have to be constantly worrying about the food that you eat for lunch. We will use some of these in the meal plans that you will see as well.

Eat What You Enjoy

Finally, the last thing to remember with your meal plan is that you ought to be enjoying the foods that are on it at all times. When you ensure that the foods that you have on your plate are those that you actually enjoy, sticking to your meal plan doesn't become such a chore, and that means that you will be able to do better as well with your own diet. Your meal plan should be loaded up with foods that you are actually excited about enjoying. Meal planning and dieting should not be a drag—you should love every moment of it!

Chapter 2: 1 Month Meal Plan

This meal plan is designed to be used for one month to help you simplify making sure that you have delicious meals to eat without having to think. These meals are fantastic options if you don't know where to start but want to enjoy your Mediterranean diet without much hassle. For each of the five weeks included, you will get one breakfast recipe, one lunch recipe, one dinner recipe, and one snack recipe to make meal planning a breeze. So, give these recipes a try! Many of them are so delicious, you'll want to enjoy them over and over again!

Week 1: Success is no accident—you have to reach for it

Mediterranean Breakfast Sandwich

Serves: 4

Time: 20 minutes

Ingredients:

- Baby spinach (2 c.)
- Eggs (4)
- Fresh rosemary (1 Tbsp.)
- Low-fat feta cheese (4 Tbsp.)
- Multigrain sandwich thins (4)
- Olive oil (4 tsp.)
- Salt and pepper according to preference
- Tomato (1, cut into 8 slices)

Instructions:

1. Preheat your oven. This recipe works best at 375° F. Cut the sandwich things in half and brush the insides with half of your olive oil. Place the things on a baking sheet and toast for about five minutes or until the edges are lightly browned and crispy.
2. In a large skillet, heat the rest of your olive oil and the rosemary. Use medium-high heat. Crack your eggs into the skillet one at a time. Cook until the whites have set while keeping the yolks runny. Break the yolks and flip the eggs until done.
3. Serve by placing spinach in between two sandwich thins, along with two tomato slices, an egg, and a tablespoon of feta cheese.

Greek Chicken Bowls

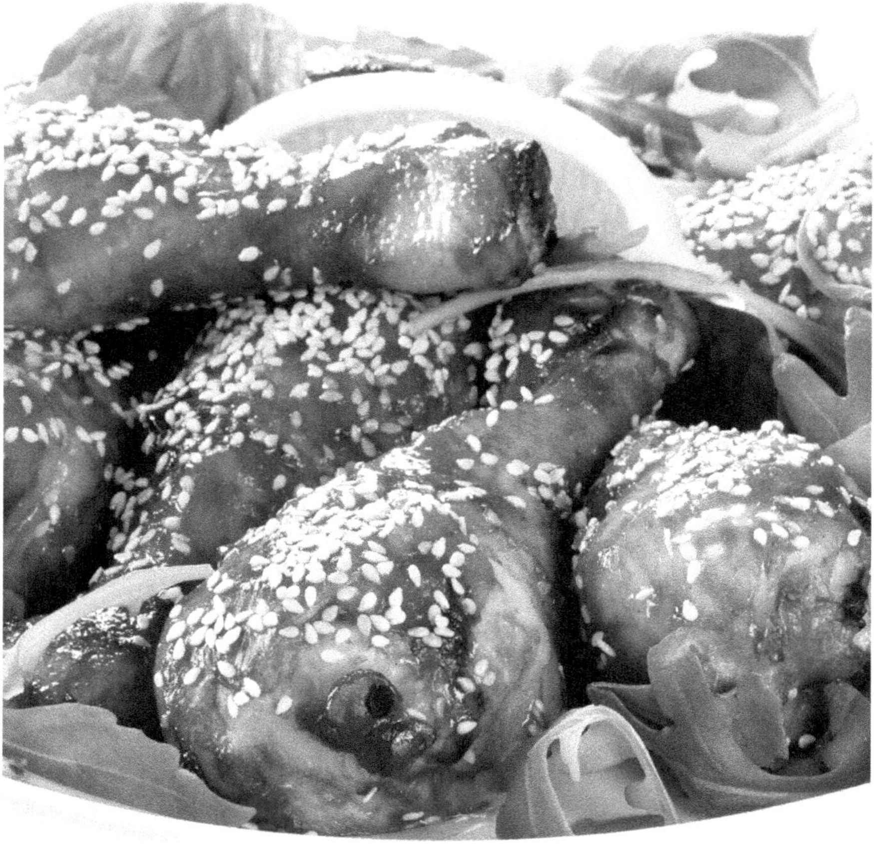

Serves: 4

Time: 20 minutes

Ingredients:

- Arugula (4 c.)
- Chicken breast tenders (1 lb.)
- Cucumber (1, diced)
- Curry powder (1 Tbsp.)
- Dried basil (1 tsp.)
- Garlic powder (1 tsp.)
- Kalamata olives (2 Tbsp.)
- Olive oil (1 Tbsp.)
- Pistachios (0.25 c., chopped)
- Red onion (half, sliced)
- Sunflower seeds (0.25 c.)
- Tzatziki sauce (1 c.)

Instructions:

1. In a bowl, mix in the chicken tenders, curry powder, dried basil, and garlic powder. Make sure to coat the chicken evenly.
2. Heat one tablespoon of olive oil over medium-high. Add the chicken and cook for about four minutes on each side. Remove from the pan and set aside to cool.
3. Place one cup of arugula into four bowls. Toss in the diced cucumber, onion, and kalamata olives.
4. Chop the chicken and distribute evenly between the four bowls.
5. Top with tzatziki sauce, pistachio seeds, and sunflower seeds.

Ratatouille

Serves: 8

Time: 1 hour 30 minutes

Ingredients:

- Crushed tomatoes (1 28 oz. can)
- Eggplants (2)
- Fresh basil (4 Tbsp., chopped)
- Fresh parsley (2 Tbsp., chopped)
- Fresh thyme (2 tsp.)
- Garlic cloves (4, minced and 1 tsp, minced)
- Olive oil (6 Tbsp.)
- Onion (1, diced)
- Red bell pepper (1, diced)
- Roma tomatoes (6)
- Salt and pepper to personal preference
- Yellow bell pepper (1, diced)
- Yellow squashes (2)
- Zucchinis (2)

Instructions:

1. Get your oven ready. This recipe works best at 375° F.
2. Slice the tomatoes, eggplant, squash, and zucchini into thin rounds and set them to the side.
3. Heat up two tablespoons of olive oil in an oven safe pan using medium-high heat. Sauté your onions, four cloves of garlic, and bell peppers for about ten minutes or when soft. Add in your pepper and salt along with the full can of crushed tomatoes. Add in two tablespoons of basil. Stir thoroughly.
4. Take the vegetable slices from earlier and arrange them on top of the sauce in a pattern of your choosing. For example, a slice of eggplant, followed by a slice of tomato, squash, and zucchini, then repeating. Start from the outside and work inward to the center of your pan. Sprinkle salt and pepper overtop the veggies.
5. In a bowl, toss in the remaining basil and garlic, thyme, parsley, salt, pepper, and the rest of the olive oil. Mix it all together, and spoon over the veggies.
6. Cover your pan and bake for 40 minutes. Uncover and then continue baking for another 20 minutes.

Snack Platter

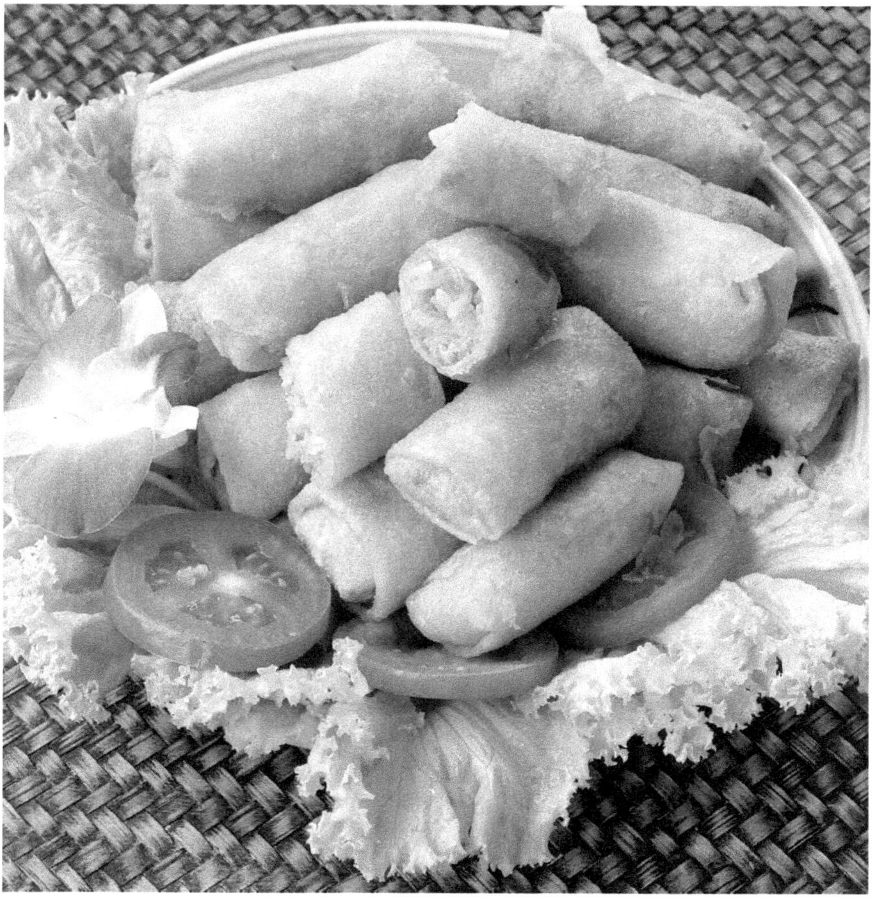

Serves: 6

Time:

Ingredients:

Rosemary Almonds

- Butter (1 Tbsp.)

- Dried rosemary (2 tsp.)
- Salt (pinch)
- Whole almonds (2 c.)

Hummus

- Chickpeas (1 15 oz. can, drained and rinsed)
- Garlic clove (1, peeled)
- Lemon (half, juiced)
- Olive oil (2 Tbsp.)
- Salt and pepper according to personal preference
- Tahini (2 Tbsp.)
- Water (2 Tbsp.)

Other sides

- Bell pepper (1, sliced)
- Cucumber (1, sliced)
- Feta cheese (4 oz, cubed)
- Kalamata olives (handful, drained)
- Pepperoncini peppers (6, drained)
- Pitas (6, sliced into wedges)
- Small fresh mozzarella balls (18)
- Soppressata (6 oz.)
- Sweet cherry peppers (18)

Instructions:

1. To get started, make your rosemary almonds. Take a large skillet and place it on a burner set to medium heat. Start melting the butter in, then toss in the almonds, rosemary and a bit of salt. Toss the nuts on occasion to ensure even coating.
2. Cook the almonds for roughly ten minutes, getting them nicely toasted. Set the almonds off to the side to let them cool.
3. Now you'll set out to make the hummus. Take a blender or food processor and toss in the hummus ingredients. Blend until you get a nice, smooth paste. If you find that your paste is too thick, try blending in a bit of water until you get the desired consistency. Once you have the right consistency, taste for seasoning and adjust as necessary.
4. Pour and scrape the hummus into a bowl and drizzle in a bit of olive oil. Set it off to the side to get the rest of the platter going.
5. Grab the sweet cherry peppers and stuff them with the little balls of mozzarella. Arrange a platter in any pattern you like. If serving for a party or family, try keeping each snack in its own little segment to keep things looking neat.

Week 2: Self-belief and effort will take you to what you want to achieve

Breakfast Quesadilla

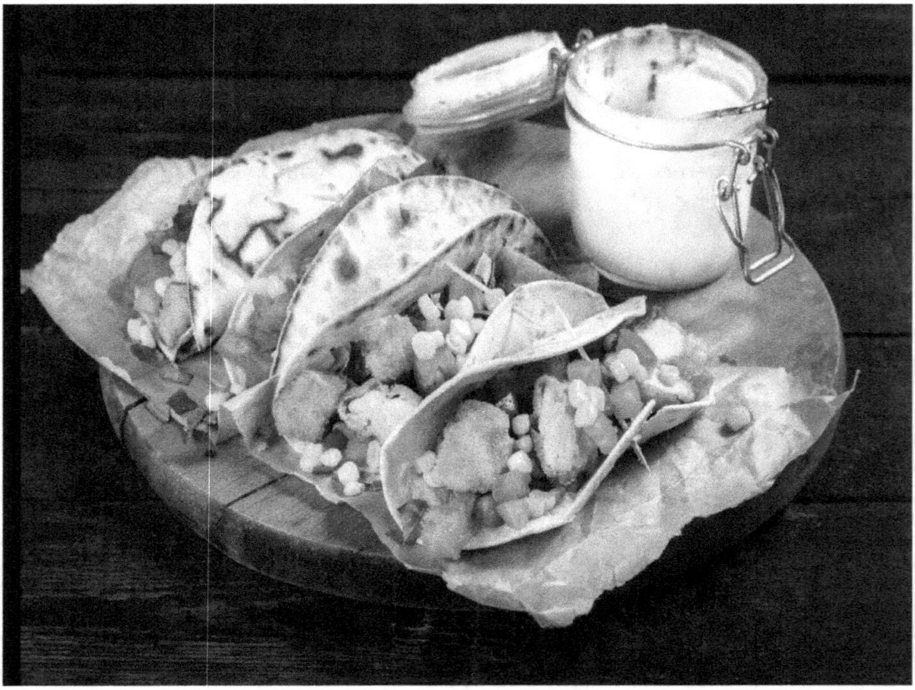

Serves: 1

Time: 10 minutes

Ingredients:

- Basil (handful)
- Eggs (2)
- Flour tortilla (1)
- Green pesto (1 tsp.)
- Mozzarella (0.25 c.)

- Salt and pepper according to personal preference
- Tomato (half, sliced)

Instructions:

1. Scramble your eggs until just a little runny. Remember, you will be cooking them further inside the quesadilla. Season with salt and pepper.
2. Take the eggs and spread over half of the tortilla.
3. Add basil, pesto, mozzarella cheese, and the slices of tomato.
4. Fold your tortilla and toast on an oiled pan. Toast until both sides are golden brown.

Greek Orzo Salad

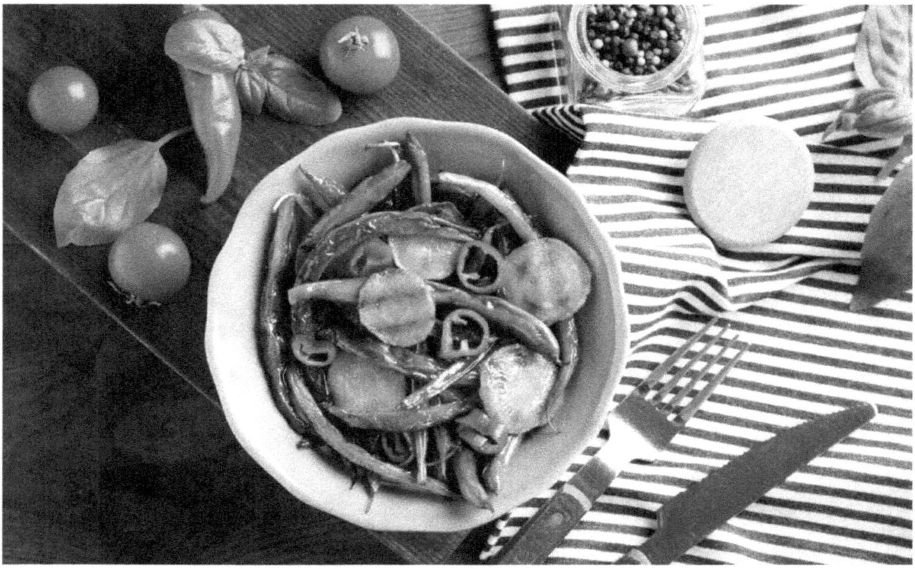

Serves: 6

Time: 25 minutes

Ingredients:

- Canned chickpeas (1 c., drained and rinsed)
- Dijon mustard (0.5 tsp)
- Dill (0.33 c., chopped)
- Dried oregano (1 tsp)
- English cucumber (half, diced)
- Feta cheese crumbles (0.5 c.)
- Kalamata olives (0.33 c., halved)
- Lemon (half, juice and zest)
- Mint (0.33 c., chopped)
- Olive oil (3 Tbsp.)
- Orzo pasta (1.25 c. when dry)
- Roasted red pepper (half, diced)
- Salt and pepper to taste
- Shallot (0.25 c., minced)
- White wine vinegar (2 Tbsp.)

Instructions:

1. Prepare the orzo according to the packaging details. Once the orzo is al dente, drain it and rinse until it drops to room temperature.
2. In a bowl, toss all the ingredients together until thoroughly incorporated.

One Pot Mediterranean Chicken

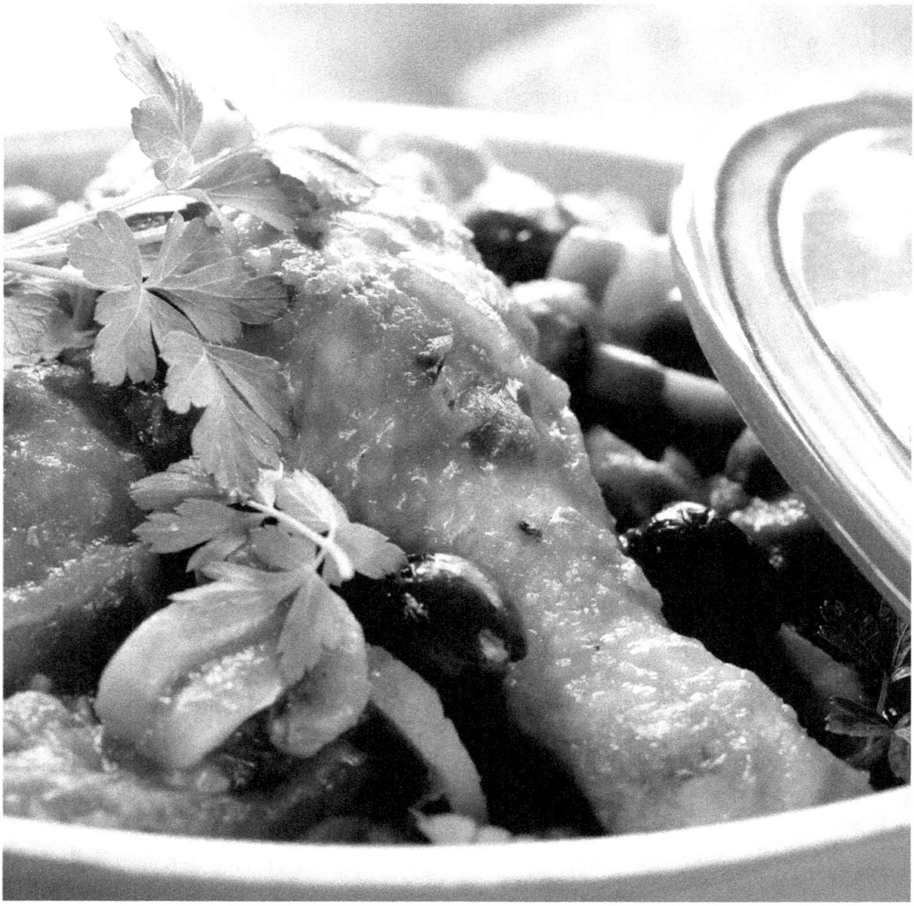

Serves: 4

Time: 1 hour

Ingredients:

- Chicken broth (3 c.)
- Chicken thighs (3, bone in, skin on)

- Chickpeas (1 15 oz can, drained and rinsed)
- Dried oregano (0.5 tsp.)
- Fresh parsley (2 Tbsp., chopped)
- Garlic cloves (2, minced)
- Kalamata olives (0.75 c., halved)
- Olive oil (2 tsp.)
- Onion (1, finely diced)
- Orzo pasta (8 ounces uncooked)
- Roasted peppers (0.5 c., chopped)
- Salt and pepper according to personal preference

Instructions:

1. Prepare your oven at 375°. Heat your olive oil in a large skillet over medium-high heat.
2. Season the chicken with salt and pepper on both sides. Toss the chicken into the skillet and cook for five minutes on each side, or until golden in color. Remove the chicken.
3. Take the skillet and drain most of the rendered fat, leaving about a teaspoon. Add the onion and cook for five minutes. Toss in the garlic and cook for an additional minute.
4. Now you will want to add the orzo, roasted peppers, oregano, chickpeas, and olives into the pan. Add in salt and pepper.
5. Place the thighs on top of the orzo and pour in the chicken broth.
6. Bring to a boil, then cover and place in the oven. Bake for 35 minutes or until chicken has cooked through. Top with parsley and serve.

Mediterranean Nachos

Serves: 6

Time: 10 minutes

Ingredients:

- Canned artichoke hearts (1 c., rinsed, drained, and dried)
- Canned garbanzo beans (0.75 c., rinsed, drained, and dried)
- Feta cheese (0.5 c., crumbled)
- Fresh cilantro (2 Tbsp., chopped)
- Pine nuts (2.5 Tbsp.)
- Roasted red peppers (0.5 c., dried)
- Sabra Hummus (half of their 10 oz. container)
- Tomatoes (0.5 c., chopped)
- Tortilla chips (roughly half a bag)

Instructions:

1. Get your oven ready by setting it to 375°F. In a baking pan, layer the tortilla chips, and spread hummus over them evenly. Top with garbanzo beans, red peppers, artichoke hearts, feta cheese, and pine nuts.
2. Bake for about five minutes or until warmed through. Remove the baking pan and top the nachos with fresh cilantro and tomatoes. Serve and enjoy.

Week 3: The harder you work, the greater the success

Breakfast Tostadas

Serves: 4

Time: 15 minutes

Ingredients:

- Beaten eggs (8)
- Cucumber (0.5 c., seeded and chopped)
- Feta (0.25 c., crumbled)
- Garlic powder (0.5 tsp)
- Green onions (0.5 c., chopped)
- Oregano (0.5 tsp)
- Red Pepper (0.5 c., diced)
- Roasted red pepper hummus (0.5 c.)
- Skim milk (0.5 c.)
- Tomatoes (0.5 c., diced)
- Tostadas (4)

Instructions:

1. In a large skillet, cook the red pepper for two minutes on medium heat until softened. Toss in the eggs, garlic powder, milk, oregano, and green onions. Stir constantly until the egg whites have set.
2. Top the tostadas with hummus, egg mixture, cucumber, feta, and tomatoes.

Roasted Vegetable Bowl

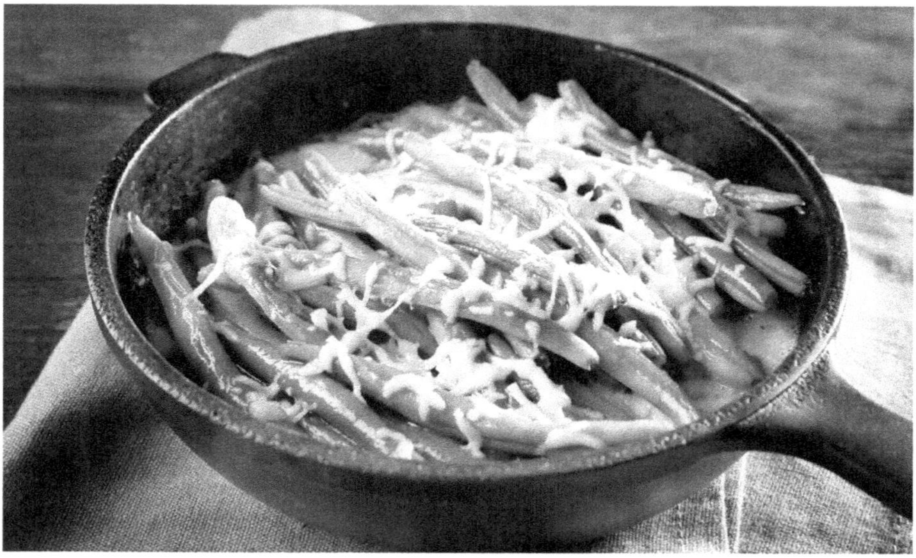

Serves: 2

Time: 45 minutes

Ingredients:

- Crushed red pepper flakes (a pinch)
- Fresh parsley (1 Tbsp., chopped)
- Kalamata olives (0.25 c.)
- Kale (1 c., ribboned)
- Lemon juice (1 Tbsp.)
- Marinated artichoke hearts (0.25 c., drained and chopped)
- Nutritional yeast (1 Tbsp.)
- Olive oil (1 Tbsp., then enough to drizzle)

- Salt and pepper to taste
- Spaghetti squash (half, seeds removed)
- Sun-dried tomatoes (2 Tbsp., chopped)
- Walnuts (0.25 c., chopped)

Instructions:

1. Get your oven ready by setting it to 400° F. Take a baking sheet and blanket it with parchment paper.
2. Take the squash half and place it on the parchment paper. Drizzle olive oil over the side that is cut, and season with salt and pepper. Turn it over so it is facing cut side down and bake for 40 minutes. It is ready when it is soft.
3. Remove the squash shell, and season with a bit more salt and pepper.
4. Stack the kale, artichoke hearts, walnuts, sun-dried tomatoes, and kalamata olives on the squash.
5. Squeeze the lemon juice over and drizzle olive oil. Finish with chopped parsley and a bit of crushed red pepper flakes.

Mediterranean Chicken

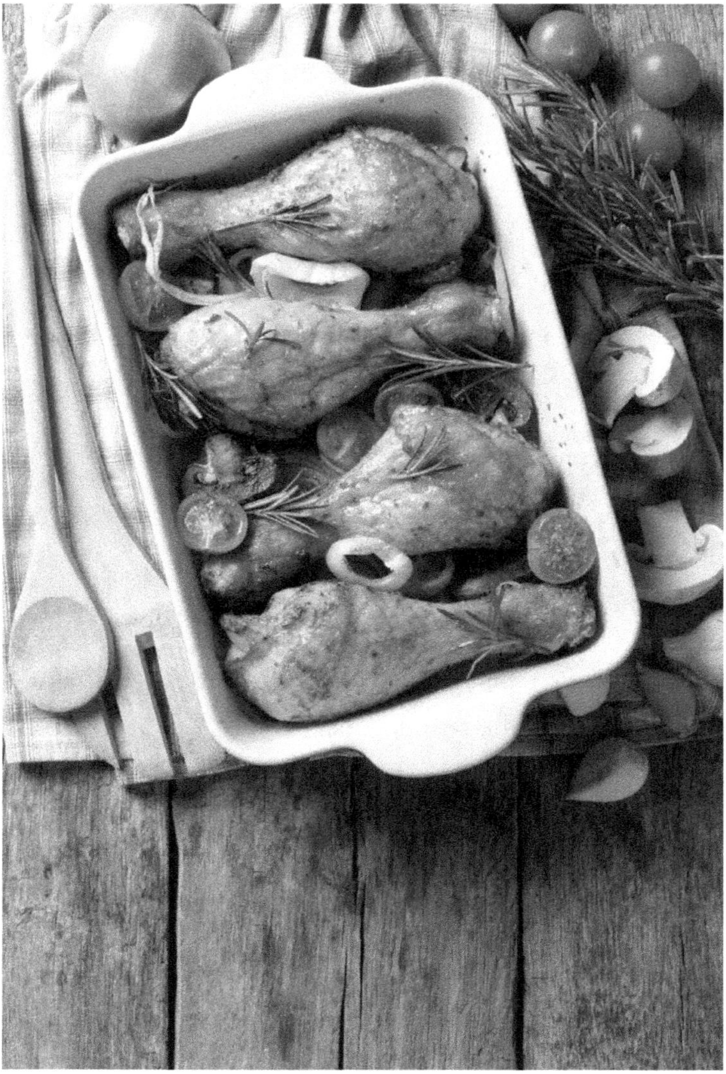

Serves: 4

Time: 40 minutes

Ingredients:

- Chicken breasts (1 lb., boneless, skinless)
- Chives (2 Tbsp., chopped)
- Feta cheese (0.25 c., crumbled)
- Garlic (1 tsp., minced)
- Italian seasoning (1 tsp.)
- Lemon juice (2 Tbsp.)
- Olive oil (2 Tbsp., and 1 Tbsp.)
- Salt and pepper according to personal preference
- Tomatoes (1 c., diced)

Instructions:

1. Pour in two tablespoons of olive oil, the lemon juice, salt, pepper, garlic, and Italian seasoning in a resealable plastic bag. Add in the chicken, seal and shake to coat the chicken.
2. Allow the chicken to marinate for at least 30 minutes in the refrigerator.
3. Heat the rest of the olive oil in a pan over medium heat.
4. Place the chicken on the pan and cook for five minutes on each side, or until cooked through.
5. In a bowl, mix the tomatoes, chives, and feta cheese. Season with salt and pepper.
6. When serving, spoon the tomato mixture on top of the chicken.

Baked Phyllo Chips

Serves: 2

Time: 10 minutes

Ingredients:

- Grated cheese (your choice)
- Olive oil (enough to brush with)
- Phyllo sheets (4)
- Salt and pepper according to personal preference

Instructions:

1. Get your oven ready by setting it to 350° F. Brush olive oil over a phyllo sheet generously. Sprinkle grated cheese and your seasoning on top.
2. Grab a second sheet of your phyllo and place it on top of the first one. Again, brush with olive oil and sprinkle cheese and seasoning on top.
3. Repeat this process with the remaining sheets of phyllo. Top the stack with cheese and seasoning.
4. Once complete, cut the stack of phyllo into bite-sized rectangles. A pizza cutter may be helpful here.
5. Grab a baking sheet and blanket it with some parchment paper. Take your phyllo rectangles and place them on the parchment paper.
6. Bake in the oven for about seven minutes or until they reach a golden color.
7. Remove them from the oven and allow them to cool before serving.

Week 4: You don't need perfection—you need effort

Mini Omelets

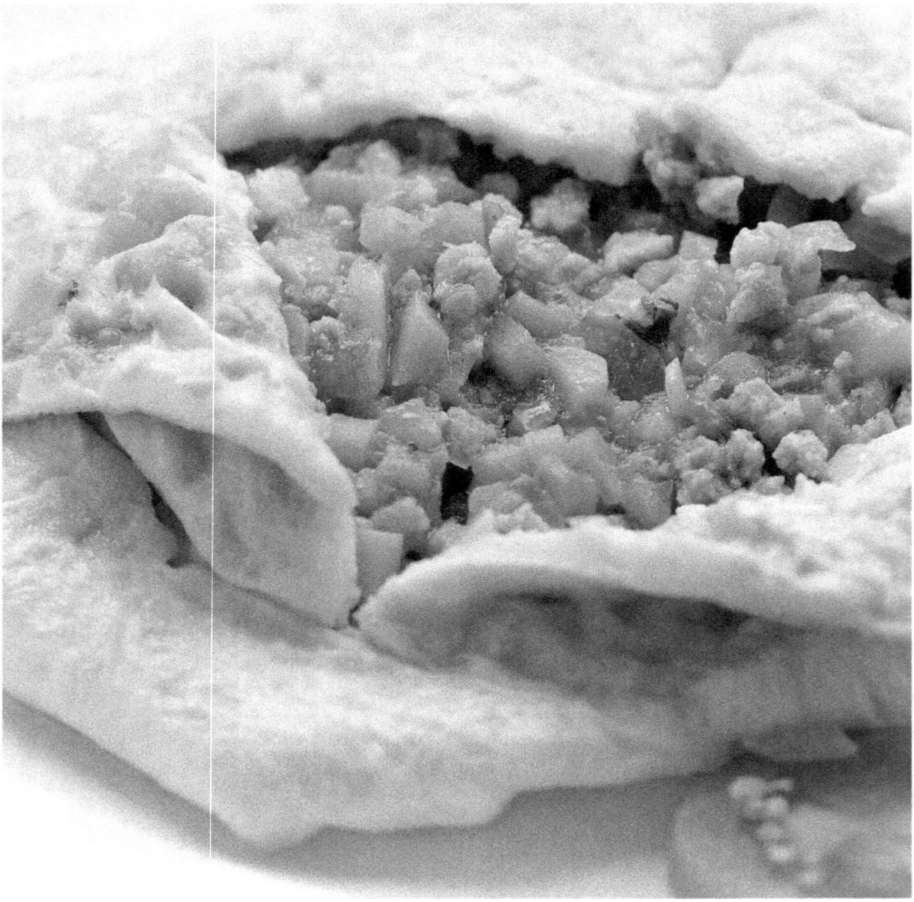

Serves: 8

Time: 40 minutes

Ingredients:

- Cheddar cheese (0.25 c., shredded)

- Eggs (8)
- Half and half (0.5 c.)
- Olive oil (2 tsps.)
- Salt and pepper according to personal preference
- Spinach (1 c., chopped)

Instructions:

1. Get your oven ready by setting it to 350° F. Prepare a muffin pan or ramekins by greasing them with olive oil.
2. In a bowl, beat the eggs and dairy until you have a fluffy consistency.
3. Stir in the cheese and your seasonings. Pour in the spinach and continue beating the eggs.
4. Pour the egg mixture into your ramekins or muffin pan.
5. Bake the omelets until they have set, which should be roughly 25 minutes. Remove them from the oven and allow them to cool before serving.

Basil Shrimp Salad

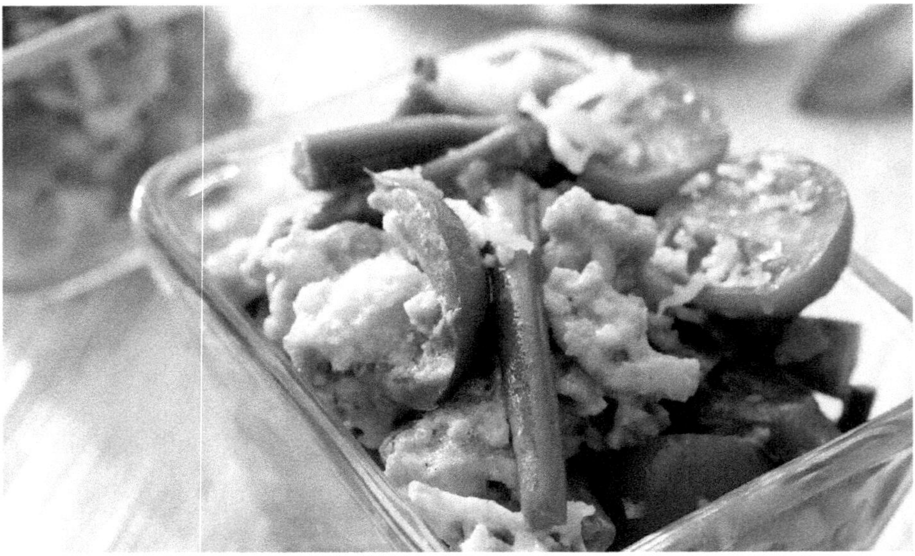

Serves: 2

Time: 40 minutes

Ingredients:

- Dried basil (1 tsp.)
- Lemon juice (1 Tbsp.)
- Olive oil (1 tsp.)
- Romaine lettuce (2 c.)
- Shrimp (12 medium or 8 large)
- White wine vinegar (0.25 c.)

Instructions:

1. Whisk together the white wine vinegar, olive oil, lemon juice, and basil. Stick your shrimp in the marinade for half an hour.
2. Take the marinade and shrimp and cook in a skillet over medium heat until cooked through.
3. Allow the shrimp to cool along with the juice and pour into a bowl. Toss in the romaine lettuce and mix well to get the flavor thoroughly infused in the salad. Serve.

Mediterranean Flounder

Serves: 4

Time: 40 minutes

Ingredients:

- Capers (0.25 c.)
- Diced tomatoes (1 can)
- Flounder fillets (1 lb.)
- Fresh basil (12 leaves, chopped)
- Fresh parmesan cheese (3 Tbsp., grated)
- Garlic cloves (2, chopped)
- Italian seasoning (a pinch)
- Kalamata olives (0.5 c., pitted and chopped)
- Lemon juice (1 tsp.)
- Red onion (half, chopped)
- White wine (0.25 c.)

Instructions:

1. Set your oven to 425° F. Take a skillet and pour in enough olive oil to sauté the onion until soft. Cook on medium-high heat.
2. Toss in the garlic, Italian seasoning, and tomatoes. Cook for an additional five minutes.
3. Pour in the wine, capers, olives, lemon juice, and only half of the basil you chopped.
4. Reduce the heat to low and stir in the parmesan cheese. Simmer for ten minutes or until the sauce has thickened.
5. Place the flounder fillets in a baking pan and pour the sauce over top. Sprinkle the remaining basil on top and bake for 12 minutes.

Nutty Energy Bites

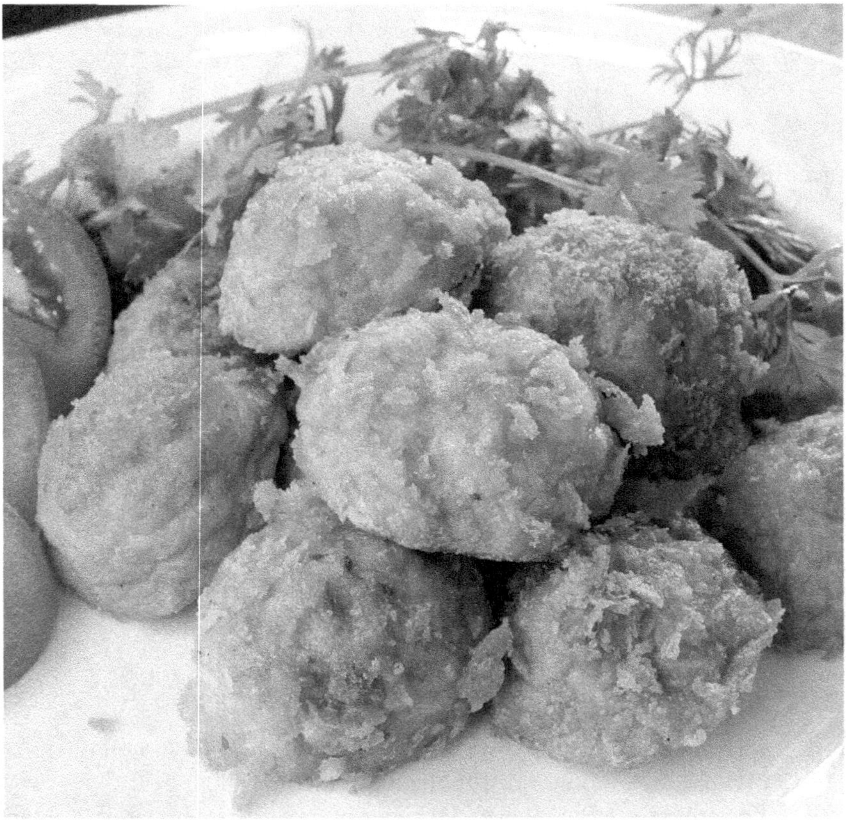

Serves: 10

Time: 10 minutes

Ingredients:

- Dried dates (1 c., pitted)
- Almonds (0.5 c.)
- Pine nuts (0.25 c.)

- Flaxseeds (1 Tbsp., milled) Porridge oats (2 Tbsp.)
- Pistachios (0.25 c., coarsely ground)

Instructions:

1. Take the dates, pine nuts, milled flaxseeds, almonds, and porridge oats and pour them into a food processor or blender. Mix until thoroughly incorporated.
2. Using a tablespoon, scoop the mixture and roll it between your hands until you have a small, bite-sized ball. Do this until you have used the entirety of the dough. This recipe should be enough for about ten.
3. On a plate, sprinkle your ground pistachios. Take the energy balls and roll them on the pistachio grounds, making sure to coat them evenly. Serve or store in the refrigerator.

Week 5: Transformation Happens One Day at a Time

Mediterranean Breakfast Bowl

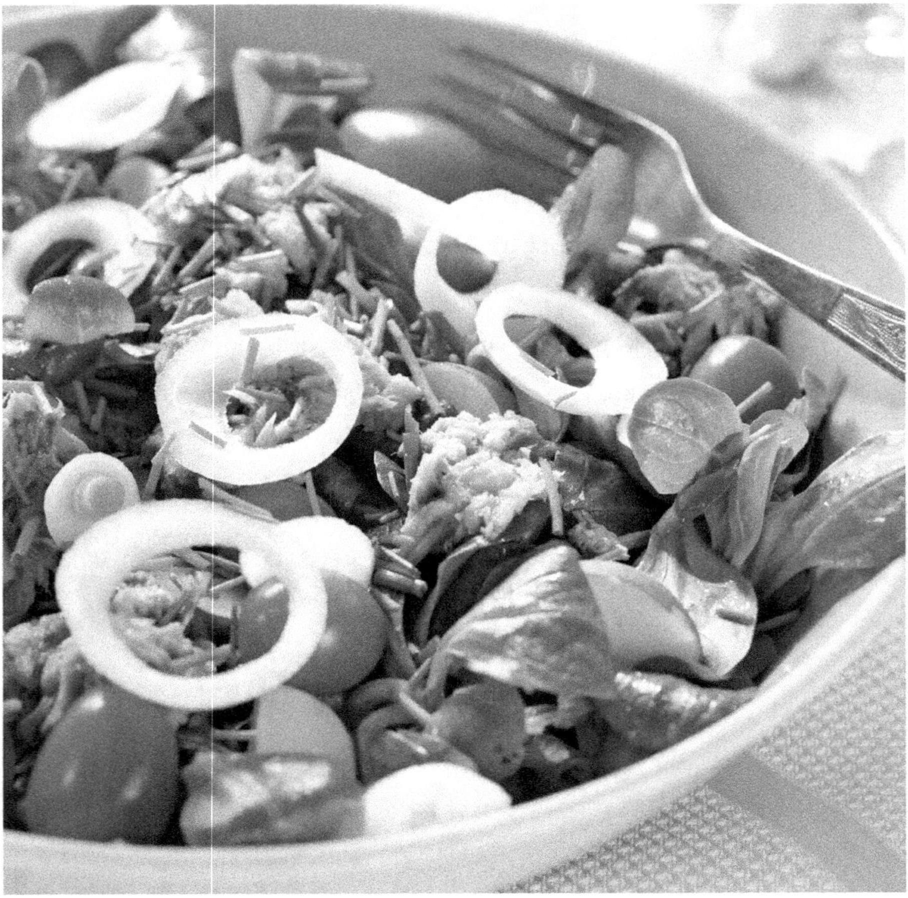

Serves: 1

Time: 25 minutes

Ingredients:

- Artichoke hearts (0.25 c., chopped)
- Baby arugula (2 c.)
- Capers (1 Tbsp.)
- Egg (1)
- Feta (2 Tbsp., crumbled)
- Garlic (0.25 tsp)
- Kalamata olives (5, chopped)
- Lemon thyme (1 Tbsp., chopped)
- Olive oil (0.5 Tbsp.)
- Pepper (0.25 tsp)
- Sun-dried tomatoes (2 Tbsp., chopped)
- Sweet potato (1 c., cubed)

Instructions:

1. Take your olive oil and, when hot, pan fry your sweet potatoes for 5-10 minutes until they have softened. Then, sprinkle on the seasonings.
2. Place arugula into a bowl, then top with potatoes, then everything but the egg.
3. Prepare the egg to your liking and serve.

Chicken Shawarma Pita Pockets

Serves: 6

Time: 40 minutes

Ingredients:

- Cayenne (0.5 tsp)
- Chicken thighs (8, boneless, skinless, bite-sized pieces)
- Cloves (0.5 tsp, ground)
- Garlic powder (0.75 Tbsp.)
- Ground cumin (0.75 Tbsp.)
- Lemon juice (1 lemon)
- Olive oil (0.33 c.)
- Onion (1, sliced thinly)
- Paprika (0.75 Tbsp.)
- Salt
- Turmeric powder (0.75 Tbsp.)

To serve:

- Pita pockets (6)
- Tzatziki sauce
- Arugula
- Diced tomatoes
- Diced onions
- Sliced Kalamata olives

Instructions:

1. Combine all spices. Then, place all chicken, already diced, into the bowl. Coat well, then toss in onions, lemon juice, and oil. Mix well and let marinade for at least 3 hours, or overnight.
2. Preheat the oven to 425 F. Allow chicken to sit at room temperature a few minutes. Then, spread it on an oiled sheet pan. Roast for 30 minutes.
3. To serve, fill up a pita pocket with tzatziki, chicken, arugula, and any toppings you prefer. Enjoy.

Turkey Mediterranean Casserole

Serves: 6

Time: 35 minutes

Ingredients:

- Fusilli pasta (0.5 lbs.)
- Turkey (1.5 c., chopped)
- Sun dried tomatoes (2 Tbsp., drained)
- Canned artichokes (7 oz., drained)
- Kalamata olives (3.5 oz., drained and chopped)
- Parsley (0.5 Tbsp., chopped and fresh)
- Basil (1 T, fresh)
- Salt and pepper to taste
- Marinara sauce (1 c.)
- Black chopped olives (2 oz., drained)
- Mozzarella cheese (1.5 c., shredded)

Instructions:

1. Warm your oven to 350 F. Prepare your pasta according to the directions, drain, and place into a bowl. Prepare your basil, parsley, olives, tomatoes, artichokes, and other ingredients.
2. Mix together the pasta with the turkey, tomatoes, olives, artichokes, herbs, seasoning, and marinara sauce. Give it a good mix to incorporate all of the ingredients evenly.
3. Take a 9x13 oven-safe dish and layer in the first half of your pasta mixture. Then, sprinkle on half of your mozzarella cheese. Top with the rest of the pasta, then sprinkle on the chopped black olives as well. Spread the rest of the shredded cheese on top, then bake it for 20-25 minutes. It is done when the cheese is all bubbly and the casserole is hot.

Heirloom Tomato and Cucumber Toast

Serves: 2

Time: 5 minutes

Ingredients:

- Heirloom tomato (1, diced)
- Persian cucumber (1, diced)
- Extra virgin olive oil (1 tsp)
- Oregano (a pinch, dried)
- Kosher salt and pepper
- Whipped cream cheese (2 tsp)
- Whole grain bread (2 pieces)
- Balsamic glaze (1 tsp)

Instructions:

4. Combine the tomato, cucumber, oil, and all seasonings together.
5. Spread cheese across bread, then top with mixture, followed by balsamic glaze.

Chapter 3: Maintaining Your Diet

Sticking to a diet can be tough. You could see that other people are having some great food and wish that you could enjoy it too. You might realize that you miss the foods that you used to eat and feel like it's a drag to not be able to enjoy them. When you are able to enjoy the foods that you are eating, sticking to your diet is far easier. However, that doesn't mean that you won't miss those old foods sometimes. Thankfully, the Mediterranean diet is not a very restrictive one—you are able to enjoy foods in moderation that would otherwise not be allowed, and because of that, you can take the slice of cake at the work party, or you can choose to pick up a coffee for yourself every now and then. When you do this, you're not doing anything wrong, so long as you enjoy food in moderation.

Within this chapter, we are going to take a look at several tips that you can use that will help you with maintaining your diet so that you will be able to stick to it, even when you feel like things are getting difficult. Think of this as your guide to avoiding giving in entirely—this will help you to do the best thing for yourself so that you can know that you are healthy. Now, let's get started.

Find Your Motivation

First, if you want to keep yourself on your diet, one of the best things that you can do is make sure that you find and stick to your motivation. Make sure that you know what it is in life that is motivating you. Are you losing weight because a doctor told you to? Fair enough—but how do you make that personal and about yourself? Maybe instead of looking at it as a purely health-related choice, look at it as something that you are doing because of yourself. Maybe you are eating better so that you are able to watch your children graduate or so that you can run after them at the park and stay healthy, even when it is hard to do so.

Remind Yourself Why You are Eating Healthily

When you find that you are struggling to eat healthily, remind yourself of why you are doing it in the first place. When you do this enough, you will begin to resist the urges easier than ever. Make it a point to tell yourself not to eat something a certain way. Take the time to remind yourself that you don't need to order that greasy pizza—you are eating better foods because you want to be there for your children or grandchildren.

Reminding yourself of your motivation is a great way to overcome those cravings that you may have at any point in time. The cravings that you have are usually strong and compelling, but if you learn to overcome them, you realize that they weren't actually as powerful as you thought they were. Defeat the cravings. Learn to tell yourself that they are not actually able to control you. Tell yourself that you can do better with yourself.

Eat Slowly

Now, on the Mediterranean diet, you should already be eating your meals with other people anyway. You should be taking the time to enjoy those meals while talking to other people and ensuring that you get that connection with them, and in doing so, you realize that you are able to do better. You realize that you are able to keep yourself under control longer, and that is a great way to defend and protect yourself from overeating.

When you eat slowly, you can get the same effect. Eating slowly means that you will have longer for your brain to realize that you should be eating less. When you are able to trigger that sensation of satiety because you were eating slowly, you end up eating fewer calories by default, and that matters immensely.

Keep Yourself Accountable

Don't forget that, ultimately, your diet is something that you must control on your own. Keep yourself accountable by making sure that you show other people what you are doing. If you are trying to lose weight, let them know, and tell them how you plan to do so. When you do this, you are able to remind yourself that other people know what you are doing and why—this is a great way to foster that sense of accountability because you will feel like you have to actually follow through, or you will be embarrassed by having to admit fault. You could also make accountability to yourself as well. When you do this, you are able to remind yourself that your diet is your own. Using apps to track your food and caloric intake is just one way that you can do this.

Remember Your Moderation

While it can be difficult to face a diet where you feel like you can't actually enjoy the foods that you would like to eat, the truth is that on the Mediterranean diet, you are totally okay to eat those foods that you like or miss if you do so in moderation. There is nothing that is absolutely forbidden on the Mediterranean diet—there are just foods that you should be restricting regularly. However, that doesn't mean that you can't have a treat every now and then.

Remembering to live in moderation will help you from feeling like you have to cheat or give up as well. When you are able to enjoy your diet and still enjoy the times where you want to enjoy your treats, you realize that there is actually a happy medium between sticking to the diet and deciding to quit entirely.

Identify the Difference between Hunger and Craving

Another great way to help yourself stick to your diet is to recognize that there is a very real difference between actually being hungry and just craving something to eat. In general, cravings are felt in the mouth—when you feel like you are salivating or like you need to eat something, but it is entirely in your head and mouth, you know that you have a craving. When you are truly hungry, you feel an emptiness in your stomach—you are able to know because your abdomen is where the motivation is coming from.

Being able to tell when you have a craving and when you are genuinely hungry, you can usually avoid eating extra calories that you didn't actually need. This is major—if you don't want to overeat, you need to know when your body actually needs something and when it just wants something. And if you find that you just want something, that's okay too—just find a way to move on from it. If you want to indulge a bit here and there, there's no harm in that!

Stick to the Meal Plan

When it comes to sticking to a diet, one of the easiest and most straightforward ways to do so is to just stick to your meal plan that you set up. You have it there for a reason—it is there for you to fall back on, and the sooner that you are willing to accept that, recognizing that ultimately, you can stay on track when you don't have to think about things too much, the better you will do. You will be able to succeed on your diet because you will know that you have those tools in place to protect you—they will be lined up to ensure that your diet is able to provide you with everything that you need and they will also be there so that you can know that you are on the right track.

Drink Plenty of Water

Another key to keeping yourself on track with your diet is to make sure that you drink plenty of water throughout the day. Oftentimes, we mistake our thirst with hunger and eat instead. Of course, if you're thirsty, food isn't going to really fix your problem, and you will end up continuing to mix up the sensation as you try to move past it. The more you eat, the thirstier you will get until you realize that you're full but still feeling "hungry." By drinking plenty of water any time that you think that you might want to eat, you will be able to keep yourself hydrated, and in addition, you will prevent yourself from unintentionally eating too much.

Eat Several Times Per Day

One of the best ways to keep yourself on track with your diet is to make sure that you are regularly eating. By eating throughout the day, making sure that you keep yourself full, it is easier to keep yourself strong enough to resist giving in to cravings or anything else. When you do this regularly, you will discover that you can actually keep away much of your cravings so that you are more successful in managing your diet.

Eating several times per day often involves small meals and snacks if you prefer to do so. Some people don't like doing this, but if you find that you're one of those people who will do well on a diet when you are never actually hungry enough to get desperate enough to break it, you will probably be just fine.

Fill Up on Protein

Another great way to protect yourself from giving in and caving on your diet is to make sure that you fill up on protein. Whether it comes from an animal or plant source, make sure that every time you eat, you have some sort of tangible protein source. This is the best way to keep yourself on track because protein keeps you fuller for longer. When you eat something that's loaded up with protein, you don't feel the need to eat as much later on. The protein is usually very dense, and that means that you get to resist feeling hungry for longer than you thought that you would.

Some easy proteins come from nuts—but make sure that you are mindful that you do not end up overeating during this process—you might unintentionally end up eating too many without realizing it. While you should be eating proteins regularly, make sure that you are mindful of calorie content as well!

Keep Only Healthy Foods

A common mistake that people make while dieting is that they end up caving when they realize that their home is filled up with foods that they shouldn't be eating. Perhaps you are the only person in your home that is attempting to diet. In this case, you may end up running into a situation where you have all sorts of non-compliant foods on hand. You might have chips for your kids or snacks that your partner likes to eat on hand. You may feel like it is difficult for you to stay firm when you have that to consider, and that means that you end up stuck in temptation.

One of the best ways to prevent this is to either cut all of the unhealthy junk out of your home entirely or make sure that you keep the off-limits foods in specific places so that you don't have to look at it and see it tempting you every time that you go to get a snack for yourself. By trying to keep yourself limited to just healthy foods, you will be healthier, and you will make better decisions.

Eat Breakfast Daily

Finally, make sure that breakfast is non-negotiable. Make sure that you enjoy it every single day, even if you're busy. This is where those make-ahead meals can come in handy; by knowing that you have to keep to a meal plan and knowing that you already have the food on hand, you can keep yourself fed. Breakfast sets you up for success or failure—if you want to truly succeed on your diet, you must make sure that you are willing to eat those healthier foods as much as possible, and you must get started on the right foot. Enjoy those foods first thing every day. Eat so that you are not ravenous when you finally do decide that it is time to sit down and find something to eat. Even if you just have a smoothie or something quick to eat as you go, having breakfast will help you to persevere.

PART III

Chapter 1: Muscle Mass

You have probably heard by now of the many benefits of having more of your body being composed of muscle mass. And yet, I'd venture to guess you still don't know the half of it!

If you're a woman, thirty percent of your body is made up of muscle mass; for men, it's around forty. The bottom line is, we all want more muscle! Muscle gives us that long and lean appearance—with nicely shaped muscles. Muscular people are viewed as healthy people. Obviously, they are also stronger. Too much fat can lead to all kinds of health problems, not to mention all the clothes you have that you can't wear!

There are many, many reasons to desire to build more muscle, but I'll give you the one that is at the top of the list for me: muscle burns fat. That's right! Muscle burns fat not only when you're in the gym or somewhere else, hitting the weights, or doing body resistance training, it does so when you're at rest. That is correct. Muscle eats away at fat while you're lolling on the sofa watching that Sunday afternoon football game.

This is why we love muscle!

Many folks don't do weight training because they think they have to head to the gym. It's a very common myth that it's necessary to use weights in order to add muscle. But it's just that—a myth. You also don't have to purchase a room full of expensive weights, gadgets and other equipment to use to build muscle at home.

I'm going to let you in on a little secret. You can build muscle using just...you. It is true. You can use your own body's resistance against itself to burn fat and build muscle. It's awesome! This way, there are no excuses. You don't have to pay a gym membership, drive yourself there, or even leave the comfort of your own home.

I'm going to give you nine different muscle-building, fat-burning workouts, and we're going to talk—just a little—about a few things you can do in the area of diet. Yes, diet. Not "diet" as in a bad word—like "I feel miserable after eating badly for the last two weeks and I need to go on a diet." Not that sort of talk. We'll simply touch on some of the foods you should be eating and some of the food you shouldn't be if you're genuinely interested in losing some weight.

Before we get into the exercises, let's cover some basics.

1.1. How Muscle is Built

Simply put in laymen's terms, when you work out, you essentially damage your muscles. Muscle tissue is broken down. When this process happens, your body gets busy repairing and replacing these damaged tissues. To get just a little technical during this process, the body has a process on the cellular level in which it repairs or replaces the damaged muscle fibers. It fuses these fibers together to form new myofibrils (muscle protein strands). Repaired myofibrils are larger in thickness and are greater in number, thus causing muscle hypertrophy (growth). This process doesn't happen when you are lifting weights, though. It happens afterward when the body is at rest. That's why rest is absolutely a key component to muscle growth. The hard work is only half the process. But fortunately the rest—pun intended—is easy.

Chapter 2: The Upper Body

"Can we please have a moment of silence for all those stuck in traffic on the way to the gym?" —Anonymous

These aren't always the easiest exercises to do—well, actually, exercising isn't exactly easy anyway, so scratch that. The great thing about upper body work is that this is where you will begin to see results first. So, for that reason, doing upper body work can be incredibly rewarding.

2.1 The Classic Push-Up

Push-ups are super easy, super basic and have been around forever. The reason they've been around forever is that they're also super effective. The key is to perform them correctly. If you don't, they become wasted effort.

2.1.1 *The proper way to do push-ups*

Get on the ground, belly down. Place your palms on the floor a shoulder width apart or slightly more. Keep your body straight as you push yourself up by extending your arms. Repeat. Make sure that your arms are lifting your body weight, not the muscles on the lower half of your body. Imagine there is a plank of wood on your back starting from your head to your feet. Make sure that your body is as straight as that plank in order to maintain correct body alignment.

2.1.2 *How many push-ups?*

That depends on the kind of shape you are in when you start. When you begin to do the push-ups, do they feel easy to you? Make sure you are performing the move deliberately—not going too fast that you're using momentum. The first time you try, do as many as you can while still keeping perfect form. Afterward, for your regular sets, do two-thirds that many. So, if you did fifteen but were tired by then and beginning to lose form, use ten as a target for your sets in the beginning.

As you get stronger, make the number higher. You want to continue to be challenged. Some people do as many as one-hundred push-ups per day. Perhaps that's something you can aim for. For the average beginner, three sets of ten are reasonable.

2.2 Chair-Dips

This is another upper-body exercise that, while in actuality, you're using your body-weight, you'll still need a chair or a bench or something similar. When I'm out running, there's a square cement planter that has an edge to it, and it works perfectly.

Dips further work the rhomboid muscles in your back and synchronize with push-ups on working your triceps.

Get a chair/bench or another object capable of supporting your body weight and of a similar height, as explained above. Stand with your back to it. Make sure that the object is sturdy enough to support your entire body weight. Lower yourself and place your palms on the front edge of the bench, fingers pointing forward. Tuck in your elbows to your sides. Maintain this position and walk just your feet slowly in front of you. Your body weight should be resting on your arms now. Deliberately bend your arms and lower yourself. Do this until the floor is parallel to your upper arms. If you're doing it right, you'll feel it in your back and also in your triceps. Simply hold for about a second and return to the starting position.

Do three sets. Determine the number of repetitions per set the exact same way as you did for the push-ups.

2.3 Diamond Push-Ups

Oh, chicken wings—and not the kind you eat. "Chicken wing" is a common term used to refer to the fat on the back of a person's upper arm as it kind of tends to sag, resulting in an unattractive "flapping in the wind" sort of scenario when you wave your arms. Nobody has time for this, people! Not when there are exercises that will blast those wings if you simply stay consistent. Almost everyone wants tight, toned arms. It's a sexy look, and it's youthful! Tight triceps can actually defy a woman's age. So don't skimp on the upper body exercises. I'm giving you three here, and all of them work your triceps, but the Diamond Push-Up works it the most of all so if you're only worried about triceps and nothing else, do this one.

Start in the push-up position, yet instead of having your hands out to the sides, place them in front of you and put them together to create a diamond shape.

Raise yourself until your legs are straight then lower yourself until you are two inches above the ground. You will feel the burn in those triceps. Embrace the burn! The burn means the move is working.

Choose your number of reps in the same manner with all of the upper body exercises.

Chapter 3: The Core

You must not ignore the importance of core work when it comes to resistance training. Your core muscles are the ones that essentially holds everything else together.

There's a very good chance that, no matter what you're doing, you're using your core. Having a weak core takes the power away from all the rest of your muscles. Your core muscles are also responsible for your balance and stability, which is huge. Your core is not one muscle; it's a complicated interconnected series of muscles which effectively include all of them except your arms and your legs. So, I reiterate. Working your core needs to be an incredibly important part of your exercise routine.

Think about your abs. Everybody seems to be concerned with their abdominal muscles. Many people want those six-pack muscles to show. Some just want to button their favorite jeans without lying on the bed.

There's a common misconception (still) that fat can be "spot-burned." This is simply not true. The general consensus is that fat leaves the body the same way it came on—gradually and kind of all over. Don't get me wrong on this; genetics do play a role in how our bodies store fat. Some people can be perfectly proportioned pretty much everywhere on their bodies and yet have large, unattractive bellies. Those people are still more the exception than the rule.

So, the bottom line is that you cannot target fat-burning. If you really want the fat to leave your body, there are three central areas that will require your attention: diet, cardio, and resistance training. Here we are focusing on the third, and a little later I'm going to give a quick overall snapshot of the importance of combining all three.

I'm going to give you three exercises for your core. This first one, known as a Plank, could actually be used as the only core exercise you do. It is that effective and, especially considering the other exercises you'll be doing with, will touch all the muscles in your core.

Now, remember what we said about abs and fat? Here's something many people simply don't realize. Underneath however much fat we happen to be carrying on our abdominal muscles, we all have a "six-pack." Those are muscles in each of our bodies. What people are trying to do when they say they're going for six-pack abs is burn the layers of fat that cover those muscles. As I said, and much to the sadness of myself and many others, you can't target that weight.

Additionally, I'm not going to include any kind of "sit-ups" in upper body work. They've been proven to not be as effective as other exercises that work the core muscles. Also, I personally think that unless your form is always perfect with a sit-up, you may be putting certain back muscles at risk.

3.1 Plank

This one is tough, but like I said, with this one exercise and all the many variations you can do with it, you can get those core muscles strong in no time.

Start with the initial push-up position. Bend your elbows to a right angle. Let your weight rest on your forearms. You might want to get a mat or something soft to use as padding between your arms and the floor. Make sure you have a timer too. The elbows need to be beneath your shoulders directly. Your body should be forming a straight line from head to heels—like a plank. Hold this position for as long as you can without injuring yourself.

Your goal should eventually be to hold it for two minutes. I said eventually for a good reason. Planks are tough. I mean, for a lot of people, a ten-second plank and they're toast. Because so many muscles are used to hold this position, if those muscles aren't strong, it simply can't happen for very long. That's also why planks are such a good indicator of how far you've come. If, when you start it takes all you have to hold a thirty-second plank, I would venture to guess that after a religiously followed routine, within eight weeks you will have worked up to the full two minutes.

Planks are great because there are many variations of them, as well. As you get stronger, try this:

- While in plank position, lift one of your legs as high as you can and hold it there for a count of thirty. Repeat on the other side.
- You can even do a side plank. Lay down on your side with your head propped on your elbow, raise your body in that position and hold it. To increase difficulty with this one, once you are in the up position, try raising your top leg and holding it in that position.

Planks can be thought of as a "Super Move." They literally work all of your muscles. In fact, if one really wanted to, one could do planks only as their resistance training (planks in all their variations, which are many) and achieve the results they're looking for.

3.2 Reverse Crunch

Okay, so I realize I just got done telling you that sit-ups, which are essentially crunches, are not good for the back muscles. In fact, one physician has said that he has seen no other cause of back injury with the highest rate as traditional crunches.

However, the reverse crunch, despite its name, does not carry the same risks and is excellent at targeting your abdominal muscles.

Here's how to do it:

- Lie down on the floor and fully extend your arms and legs to the sides. Put your palms on the floor. Your arms should actually stay in one place as you perform the entire exercise.
- This is the position you will start from: your legs will be pulled up which will make your thighs form a right angle with the floor. You will want your feet together and also parallel to the floor.
- Move your legs towards your torso. At the same time, roll your pelvis backward. Raise your hips above the floor. The goal is to have your knees touching your chest.
- Hold this position for around a second, then lower back to the starting position.

Again, depending on your ability when you start, gauge the number of reps and sets by how they feel to your body and how hard it is for you to do them at first. Just make sure not to overestimate yourself too much. Muscle soreness from overdoing it is no fun!

3.3 Mountain Climber

Get into the top of the push-up position. This is the starting position.

Keeping your back in a straight line, bring your right knee toward your chest. Quickly bring it back to the starting position. Do the same for the left knee. Repeat but speed up the movement, alternating legs quickly as if you were running in place with your hands on the ground.

As far as how many sets, this move isn't exactly structured that way so use seconds to guide you. Try the move until you are really struggling to continue (you'll likely be out of breath) then use two-thirds of those seconds, call it a set, and do three.

Chapter 4: The Lower Body

Working out your lower body is not to be taken lightly or skimped on when doing resistance training. One particular reason for this is because your lower body contains the largest muscle in your entire body: the gluteus maximus.

Not only do most of us like to work out this muscle because it makes us "look" better, it's also a powerhouse. This muscle, along with other gluteal muscles, is one of the great stabilizers of the human body. Keeping these muscles strong can minimize aches and pains in your lower back and hips. The muscles also give you the power you need to do simple things like walk, run, and climb.

So, whenever lower body resistance training is discussed, there are two moves that are practically givens. No, it's not because they're both somewhat torturous—it's because they are effective!

When you're doing your workout, never forget the old adage, "Pain is temporary…(fill in the blank)." Usually, people say, "pain is temporary, quitting lasts forever."

That doesn't exactly apply here, but the point is that if you aren't going to be able to tolerate a little bit of pain, you aren't going to get the same results. Workouts can hurt. Muscles burn. Sometimes by the end of a good workout, you feel like you're about to croak. As far as I'm concerned, those are the very best kind! It means you've really kicked some gluteal maximuses and made some progress for the day. You have to maintain a good attitude if you're going to embark on this journey. Results don't happen overnight, but relatively you will start to see them very quickly (although, in general people who are close to you will notice before you do.) However, nothing is more satisfying than when you do look in the mirror and see results that can't be denied, or when you put on a pair of jeans that has been an eternity since they were last wore and they button easily. It's a powerful feeling.

So, here they come, the not-always-fun but ever-so-productive lower body movements.

4.1 The Lunge

If you've ever done them, you're probably feeling the burn simply at the thought! When executed correctly, these babies do burn, but they are incredibly effective.

Lunges produce fast results. You will notice that your legs and derriere are more toned and attractive looking. You will feel that you're stronger and you'll notice the difference when you do cardio—assuming you do, of course.

Lunges do not require weights, although weights can be added later on to increase the difficulty as you get into better shape.

Form in lunges is very important. The same is true with all of these exercises. If you're going to put in the effort, you may as well make sure you're doing it right in order to maximize your results.

Following is how to execute a perfect lunge:

- Stand upright and keep your body straight. Pull your shoulders back and relax your chin. Keep your chin pointed forward, don't look down. Make sure the muscles in your core are tight and engaged.
- If it helps you with balance, you can use something you have on hand, like, say, a broom. Hold it crossways in front of you and let it lightly rest on your shoulders.
- Pick a leg. Step forward using that leg. Lower your hips until both your knees are forming a right angle. Make sure that your lowered knee isn't touching the floor and that your forward knee is directly above your angle and not too far forward. Make sure that your weight is in your heels as you push yourself back up to the starting position.

- When you do push back up to the starting position, really place extra emphasis on engaging your gluteus maximus. Deliberately use the strength in that muscle to push yourself upright.

Now. Repeat. How many times? I recommend starting with three sets of ten perfectly executed lunges. If you don't feel "the burn" add a couple, or go ahead and use a barbell if you have one and put some weight on it. You can even do lunges in reverse, to vary things up.

4.2 Squat

Ah, the squat. If you haven't done them, you've probably heard of them if you have any friends at all who work out. Like lunges, they are simple, easy to execute, and incredibly effective at increasing muscle mask and making you stronger.

Also, like lunges, there are quite a few variations to squats that you can use as you get more fit. For now, of course, we'll focus on the simple squat. Again, form is super important.

Stand with your feet at least shoulder-width apart. If you feel more comfortable, it's okay to place your feet a bit wider apart. As you stand, you should focus on having your weight on your heels. Extend your arms straight out. The first thing you'll do is thrust your hips back slightly as though you are about to take a seat. Then, lower yourself down like that as if you are actually about to sit down. You'll want to go as low as you can. The goal is to make your knees bent so that your legs are parallel to the floor, again almost if you were sitting in a chair. Control your knees so they don't move forward over your feet.

The next step is simply to stand up, and when you are coming upright, squeeze your glutes at the top of the movement. So, essentially, squats are like sitting in an invisible chair, then standing up using your glutes to propel you. Very easy but super effective!

4.3 The Bridge

The bridge is another great one for strengthening your glutes and legs. Remember, before you even see the results of these exercises, you'll be stronger for doing them. And, if you eat right and take in enough protein (building blocks for muscle) you will increase the size of your muscle and consequently burn fat. So when you're doing these not-so-fun-at-the-time moves, keep that in mind!

Here's how to do a bridge: Lie on the floor, flat as a pancake. Place your hands on your sides and bend your knees. Your feet should be about shoulder-width apart. Lift your hips off the floor, using your heels to push. Keep your back straight while doing this! Hold the position for a second and squeeze those glutes.

Slowly lower back to the position you started from.

For the number of reps, use the method we discussed previously. The first time you try the exercise, go until you really feel the burn—until it's very tough to continue or until you would not be able to. However many reps that is (say it's fifteen) subtract one-third of that number and start from there.

For variety, this exercise can be performed with one leg at a time.

Chapter 5: Putting it all Together

People have different preferences in how they like to work out. To see good results from strength training, you need to work each muscle group no less than two times per week. Three times is fine and you may see faster results that way. Depending on what you want to accomplish, generally, three times is enough.

The idea is to give each muscle group a rest day in between your workouts. So people go about the entire construct differently. Some like to work their entire body in one session, then rest for a day or two and do it again, up to three times a week.

Others prefer to break the muscle group workouts up. Legs one day, arms the next, core the next, like that.

In my opinion and in consideration of the research I've done, any of the above-mentioned ways to go about it will be just as effective as another. Of course, the most important component is that it gets done.

I'd like to take a moment at the time to talk about cardiovascular workouts. I know, I know, boo, hiss. A lot of people really aren't that big on cardio. However, there's a lot to be said for a good cardio sweat session. For one thing, cardiovascular exercise improves the health of our heart and lungs. That alone should be reason enough to work some in. Also, this type of exercise, depending on the type you choose, can burn an awful lot of calories. Remember, any calories burned will contribute to that sleek, muscular look. For the muscles to come out, the fat has to come off.

Cardiovascular exercise has also been proven to affect our moods in a positive way (the same can be said for weight training.)

The best, most well-rounded exercise plans include a mixture of both. Supposing you hate cardio, you will do yourself no harm by keeping it to a minimum. The general recommendation right now is to get thirty minutes of cardio on "most" days of the week.

Given that, as an example, you could do your weights on Monday, cardio Tuesday, weights Wednesday, Cardio Thursday, weights Friday and guess what? Take the weekend off!

This is just one example of how this can all be done. You can be as creative as you want to be or as you need to be to get around a work schedule.

You could do, for instance, cardio in the morning and resistance training at night. You could work in all or part of your resistance training during your lunch hour at work.

There are no limits to the options available, so that simply means *no excuses.*

No equipment or anything fancy is required for the cardio portion either. Walking is cardio. Just walk fast enough to get your heart rate up, break a sweat and breathe a little heavy. Increase intensity as your fitness level improves.

Here's a sample plan, if you need one. I'm going to use ten reps as a standard while performing the strength training for the sake of simplicity.

Monday Morning Before Work:

Three sets of ten of each of the following:

- Push-ups
- Chair-Dips
- Diamond Push-ups

Honestly, this should take you no more than ten minutes.

Monday Lunch:

- Walk for thirty minutes

Monday Evening:

Perform three sets of the following:

- Squats
- Lunges
- Bridges
- Planks
- Mountain Climber
- Reverse Crunch

Starting out, repeat this same routine on Wednesdays and Fridays. Try this for a few weeks (or another plan of your own design) and see how it works with your schedule.

On the days that you don't walk for thirty-minutes on your lunch, per your official "schedule," do it anyway. If not that, jump on the trampoline with your little ones at night for half an hour. Ride your bike. Swim. Ski if you live near snow and/or if it's wintertime. Snow Show. Or...head to the gym. Do the elliptical or the stair-climber for half of an hour. It's really not hard to get in the minimum amount of cardio and depending on your goals, and who says you have to stop with the minimum?

If you stick to this program, you're going to see some results and you'll see them pretty quickly.

Here's another tip: throw away your scale. Okay, well you don't have to throw it away. I just don't recommend weighing yourself all the time. It could discourage you in fact, for the simple reason that muscle actually does weigh more than fat. You might gain in the beginning, and no one wants to start a workout program only to see the numbers on the scale go up. No way! Instead of worrying about the scale, judge your progress by—most importantly—how you feel, and as for changes in your body, you can always take some initial measurements and then re-measure once a week. What has always worked best for me is simply to gauge how my clothes fit. That's the biggest tell of all. I have a pair of jean shorts I'm wearing right now. A couple of months ago I couldn't get them to even think about zipping! That's the only kind of progress I need. To me, numbers on the scale don't mean a whole lot.

Chapter 6: On Your Diet

It wouldn't be right to talk about gaining muscle and losing fat without talking a bit about diet.

I'm not going to go overboard but there are a few things I'd like to touch on.

First off, as I previously spoke about at the end of chapter four—the scale—I forgot to mention another reason I don't care to use them. Most of them have a tendency to fluctuate as much as five pounds in less than twenty-four hours. In other words, if I'm going by the scale, I often will have "gained" five pounds from when I got up to when it's time for bed.

Not cool.

Not possible, either. Our bodies are made up of an estimated sixty-five percent water. It is normal for the amount of water in our bodies to fluctuate all the time. Losing water weight does not equate to losing fat. However, while we are trying to lose weight, and while we're working out, it is especially important to keep our bodies hydrated.

There are as many theories on the web as you could click on about how much water to drink, but for questions like these, I like to refer to the Mayo Clinic website, because I know that the information they put out there has been thoroughly researched. What follows is their advice on water intake:

Every single day, you lose water by breathing, sweating, urinating, and pooping. To function properly, your body's water must be replenished through the consumption of food and beverages.

The average healthy man who lives in a temperate climate needs 15.5 cups or 3.7 liters of fluids every day, and the average healthy woman living in the same place needs 11.5 cups or 2.7 liters every day.

This is about what I do for myself in a normal day and it seems to work. Regardless, don't skimp on the water.

There's another important factor when it comes to building muscle and that is protein. If you are serious about adding some muscle mass, you're going to need to eat your protein. That doesn't mean it has to be meat; there are plenty of non-meat options for protein intake. Of course, if you are a vegetarian you already know that.

Another little tip: your body needs fat to lose fat. Sounds strange, doesn't it? But if your body is starved of nutrients, it will begin to hold on to everything it has instinctually, and as a result, you won't see any weight loss.

There are a million types of "diets" out there, and this is not a book about diets so I'm not going to delve into them. If I were going to say anything at all about your diet (and don't get me wrong, your diet IS important,) I would say two words: eat clean.

What does that mean? Since clean is the opposite of dirty, in this case, think dirty equals "processed."

Do your body a giant favor and stay away from processed foods! Eat foods that are as "close" to the earth as you can.

- Lean proteins (including fish and non-meat proteins)
- Tons—and I do really mean tons—of vegetables
- Lean fat (avocado, almonds, coconut oil)
- Dairy (full-fat; eat sparingly)
- Fruits (sparingly)

It's that simple. No "TV Dinners." No boxes of macaroni and cheese, please. Nothing that has a "bunch" of ingredients, many of which you aren't even familiar with. Those are bad. Leave them in the store.

If you have a sweet tooth, indulge it, but rarely, and even a sweet tooth can be indulged in a healthy manner. There's nothing wrong with eating some strawberries topped with full fat whipped cream. Yummy!

Well, there you have it. You really are set. Everything is explained and condensed for you.

Start your weight training and your cardio, eat clean, drink your water and reap the rewards.

Go get 'em!

PART IV

CHAPTER ONE

A WARNING

Everybody is different, making every habit different. That means that all these tips coming up are subjective. It's not something that will work for everybody. Another thing you need to be aware of is that your habit could be something more. I'm going to go over this possible problem quickly. Keep in mind this is not to cure or diagnose you with anything. If you think you may have a psychological disorder, as opposed to a bad habit, please seek medical attention.

For your information, a habit is defined as a settled or regular tendency or practice; especially one that is hard to give up.

OCD, obsessive compulsive disorder, can be confused as a habit. OCD can fall into four main categories;

- checking
- contamination/mental contamination
- hoarding

- ruminations/intrusive thoughts

OCD is diagnosed by when obsessions and compulsions:

- Consume excessive amounts of time
- Causes significant distress
- Interferes with daily functions

Your habit, itself, could be OCD, or your inability to break the habit, could be caused by OCD. An example of OCD being the habit would be hoarding. An example of OCD interfering your ability to break a habit would be intrusive thoughts. Now, when breaking a habit you will have intrusive thoughts, but they should just come and go. If your intrusive thoughts are constant and interfere with your life, then OCD could be a factor.

Other psychological disorders that could be confused with a habit are, eating disorders. Anorexia nervosa and bulimia nervosa are common eating disorders where people end up starving themselves or binging and purging. A lesser known eating disorder, which is the one most likely to be confused as a habit, is a binge-eating disorder.

With binge-eating disorder, people lose control of their eating habits. Unlike with bulimia nervosa, periods of binges are not followed by purging, which is why most people with binge-eating disorder are overweight. It is the top eating disorder in the US. Symptoms of binge-eating disorder are:

- Eating an unusually large amount of food in a specific amount of time
- Eating even when you're full or not hungry
- Eating fast during binge episodes
- Eating until you are uncomfortably full
- Eating alone or in secret to avoid embarrassment
- Feeling distressed, ashamed, or guilty when not eating
- Frequent dieting, possibly without weight loss

Chances are everybody can say that they have experienced one or more of these symptoms. For example, most holidays' people will over eat. That does not mean you have binge-eating disorder. Keep in mind disorders interrupt your everyday life, and happen constantly. If you just overeat when watching TV, or when you're bored, then you probably don't have a disorder. If you are concerned that you might, then please seek medical advice.

Make sure that if you think you have a disorder to see your doctor make sure. It's better to believe you have a disease than go around with an undiagnosed disorder. I want to make sure that you can live the life you deserve and making sure that your habit isn't something more serious is important.

CHAPTER TWO

A HISTORY OF HABITS

Imagine this; your alarm goes off. You slide out of bed and slump your way to the bathroom. You do your business and then hop in the shower. Once finished you brush your teeth before you get dressed. Once dressed you head to the kitchen to have your coffee and breakfast. Now, what just happened? You were on complete autopilot. You are so used to doing the same thing every morning you don't have to think about it. That is what a habit is.

Human beings are creatures of habit. We get into a routine, and we stick to it. Then it becomes a struggle to change.

Chances are your habits are caused by stress or boredom. You start doing things to distract your brain from the stress or boredom, giving you brain a brief moment of utopia.

Stress and boredom aren't just triggers for certain habits. They're triggers for most habits. Whether you have a problem with eating, smoking, biting your nails, or spending mindless hours on the computer, whatever it may be you're using the habit to suppress those emotions. There is a chance that a deeper issue causes the stress or boredom that is being felt.

Ask yourself, is there a belief or a reason you're holding onto this habit?

The key to overcoming a habit is to figure out what is causing it. Did something happen when you were younger? Do you believe something bad is going to happen if you stop?

That's why there is no one solution. Take the habit of smoking. According to the World Health Organization, more than one billion people smoke. Most of those people are smoking for different reasons. Some may smoke because they saw their parents smoke, or their friends. They may have started smoking as a way to cope with stress.

A Loop

Every habit begins with a psychological pattern. The habit loop is a three-part process. It begins with a trigger. The trigger tells you brain to go into automatic mode and let a behavior happen. The second part is the routine which is the actual habit itself. The last part is the reward.

The reward is something your brain likes and helps it remember the loop in the future.

According to neuroscientists, habit-making behaviors are controlled in the basal ganglia. The basal ganglia are also the area of the brain that controls emotions, memories, and patterns. As stated above, a habit is a pattern.

Decisions are controlled in the prefrontal cortex. A habit starts as a behavior or decision, but the more you do it, the less the brain works. The decision-making part of your brain goes to sleep. That's what makes multitasking possible.

Good habits are programmed the same as bad habits are. A good habit, such as brushing your teeth, gets programmed by repetition just like smoking. Or learning to parallel park works the same as overeating.

The fact that they work the same is a good thing. That makes it easier for you to retrain your brain.

Problems

There are going to be problems when trying to break a habit, especially if your habit involves any stimulant. At that point, you're not just trying to stop the habit, but also working through the detox symptoms. For example, nicotine, via tobacco, is one of the most heavily consumed drugs in the world. In Australia, smoking is one of the biggest causes of, preventable, death, killing about 15,000 people per year. It's also one of the hardest to quit. Withdrawal from nicotine can cause insomnia, irritability, anxiety, and difficulty concentrating.

Slip-ups are inevitable, but if you're working to break a habit that involves any stimulating drug, it's going to be a lot harder. This could include smoking, drinking, even coffee. Keep this in the back of your mind so that you are prepared.

CHAPTER THREE

A HABITS HABITAT

Necessarily true. You can control your habits, but your environment plays a huge part of what you do on a daily basis. One of your brain's primary functions is to find and use patterns as shortcuts to process the information we're presented with on a daily basis.

In a study conducted on habits vs. intentions, researchers found that students that switched Universities were more likely to change their daily habits. Those habits were easier to change than they were for the control group because they weren't exposed to familiar daily cues. This can be seen in every bad habit that somebody has.

Eating Habits

Have you ever been driving home from work, not thinking about food, when you see your favorite fast food joint, and suddenly your start craving a cheeseburger? It's not your fault. Everybody experiences moments like that.

Our food environment is broken down into two categories; the atmosphere we encounter when eating, and how food is portioned. The cues vary from what's being eaten, its packaging or utensil size, and the amount of food. Think about when you eat out. You will undoubtedly receive a huge plate of food. You don't think you can eat it all, but then you end up cleaning your plate. Seeing an empty plate signals satiety in our brains.

Maybe eating at home will help you avoid these triggers. Not so fast. Home plate sizes have increased 22% over the last century. Where you store your food also plays a large part in your eating habits, bringing new meaning to "Out of sight, out of mind."

Don't worry though. There are ways to overcome these triggers.

- First, choose smaller plates to use at home. It takes less food to fill up a small plate. You're eating less, but you're still cleaning your plate and making your brain happy.

- Another way is to pre-portion your food. Have everything portioned out into single servings.

- It also helps to focus on one thing at a time. When you're eating, only concentrate on eating. Try not to watch TV or the computer while you're eating.

- Most importantly learn the true signs of hunger and avoid mindless eating. This comes in handy when you're not in control of the food.

Smoking Habits

Environmental triggers for smokers can be harder to break than triggers for overeaters. According to the American Psychological Association is in an area associated with smoking can cause a smoker to have a craving. That means they could walk into a bar where there are no cigarettes, ashtrays, or other smokers, yet still, have a craving because they associate the setting with smoking.

Your regular daily routine could also cause triggers. Some people associate their morning cup of coffee with smoking. An easy fix for that is to keep yourself busy in the morning. Try to distract yourself from the craving. You can also trade your coffee out for tea or juice.

Most smokers smoke while driving making the car another common trigger. If you have cravings whenever you drive try singing along to the radio or a CD. You could also substitute smoking with chewing gum while driving.

Stress is another major trigger for smokers. Cigarettes have thousands of chemicals in them that trick your brain into thinking that they are helping relieve your stress. The key to overcoming the stress trigger is to find new ways to relieve your stress. Meditation and yoga are both good stress management techniques.

Drinking Habits

Stress and anxiety are big triggers for drinking. As I mentioned earlier, they are also the cause for most habits.

There are two main types of triggers; external and internal. External are people, places, or things that trigger you desire to drink. They are easier to avoid than internal triggers. Internal triggers are, as the name states, inner emotions that trigger your desire to drink.

A good way to figure out exactly what causes your triggers is to track them for a week. Keep a journal with you and every time you have the urge to drink, write down what happened or where you were that caused the urge.

Some simple ways to avoid external triggers are to keep little, to no alcohol, at home. Socially, try avoiding situations that involve drinking. You may feel guilty turning down invitations to go out with your friends, but just remember it's not forever. You only have to turn them down until your urges become more manageable.

It won't be possible to stay away from all triggers. Always remind yourself why you are making this change. Keep a list somewhere on your person that you can read when you have the urge to drink. Talk to an accountability partner. That's what they're there for. Distract yourself. Find something to do to keep your mind off your urge. Lastly, you could also ride it out. Problem the hardest, but tell yourself that it's only temporary. That the feeling will pass.

Using your Triggers

You can also use your triggers for good. Task association is a good way to control your triggers. For instance, doctors have helped insomniacs by telling them to only go to bed when they are sleepy. If they can't sleep, they are told to go to a different room that way their bed is only associated with sleep. This could work to cut back on environmental triggers.

Instead of keeping snacks close to your work area, keep them in the kitchen or break room. That way you associate your desk with working and not with eating. Train yourself to associate your car with singing along with the radio instead of smoking. Only eat at the kitchen table and not on the couch. That way the couch is only for watching TV and the kitchen table is for eating.

CHAPTER FOUR

A SIMPLE BREAK

I'm going to start with the most basic three steps of breaking a bad habit. I don't want to overload you with a bunch of information. These first three basic steps will give you the building blocks to move onto more in-depth information.

The first step you have to take in breaking a habit is the decision to break the habit. You're probably thinking, "Duh," but you have to make sure you have a reason. If you don't have a reason to quit, you will not quit. You won't get anywhere if you go at this thinking you "might" have something you need to change. You have to know and want to change. Make a list of the reasons why you want to stop. If you can't think of anything, make a list of the bad things that will happen if you don't stop. For example, if you don't stop binge eating you could become overweight and develop serious health problems.

The next step is to be ready to face your boredom or emotions. As mentioned before habits are formed out of boredom or stress. You have to be willing to take a look at your life and figure out how to change what is causing your dissatisfaction. You must be ready to face the discomfort. We as humans don't like discomfort, but if you can overcome that, then you have surpassed one of the biggest hurdles. Make your life the way you want it to be.

The last step is to find a new way to relieve stress. You could have the life of your dreams, but you still suffer from stress. You feel stressed, so you turn to alcohol. You drink, and then you don't feel stressed. That makes you think you have everything together. Instead, you need to replace you drinking with something new, something healthy. You could use meditation or exercise as a healthy alternative.

The first three steps are:

1. Make sure you have a good reason to break your habit
2. Be ready to face the emotions and boredom that is causing your habit
3. Find a new way to handle your stress

Starting with these three steps will put you well on your way to breaking your bad habit. In the coming chapters, I will go into more detail on how to switch out your bad habits for new healthy habits.

A Big Break

As learned in the last chapter, there are three necessary steps to breaking habits. While those three steps are paramount there are other tips and tricks to take your habit breaking to the next level. We'll discuss several of them in this chapter, and flesh out even more throughout the rest of the book. A big part of break a bad habit is replacing it with a new one; I'll wait until later to explain how to start said new habit. Now, let's look at some tips to kick those habits to the curb.

1. Set a Start Date

Mark it on your calendar when you want to start changing your habit. You have to be serious about this, so having a countdown will help you to stay on track. The countdown will help to create excitement. Just like a child counting down the 25 to Christmas, or the days before their birthday. You want to drastically change your life for the better, so there should be an element of excitement.

2. Bait and Switch

Once you know what habit you want to change then, you can sub a new habit, temporary or permanent, in its place. If you're a nail-biter, try subbing in gum. Gum can also be used to help with smoking urges.

3. Discover your triggers

Knowing why we make certain decisions is the key to conquering your habits. Often we perform the habit without even realizing we're doing it. That's why it's called a habit. For a long time after my Dad quit smoking, every time he got in the car he would roll down the window and fiddle with his pocket because that's what he would do when he smoked. He never even realized he was doing that until we told him. But you can fix that by being consciously aware of when you perform your habit. There are five main triggers for habits; location, time, emotional state, other people, and an immediately preceding action. Start to take notes whenever you perform the bad habit. Soon you will be able to figure out what is triggering your problem.

4. Don't go cold turkey

Everybody has probably tried to give up something cold turkey. Cold turkey is a favorite of smokers, but it rarely ever works. It's similar to telling a child to not do something, and that will be exactly what they go and do. Cold turkey is centered on perfection. People think that they if they slip up then they have failed. Nobody is perfect. Cold Turkey leaves no wiggle room, and with something like this, you need a little wiggle room.

5. Switch up your environment

You don't have to move or do anything drastic. The smallest change can switch your brain's thinking. You always smoke in the parking lot at work; the parking lot becomes a trigger. If you change your routine just slightly you will trick your brain into not craving a cigarette. You can also use the 20-second rule. Make it so that it takes 20 more seconds for you to make your habit. If you smoke, keep your cigarettes in a draw where you have to walk to get them. If you have a problem with snacking, put your snacks in the back of the pantry.

6. Make it incremental

The best way to make a change is to set daily incremental changes. You need to wean yourself off of you habit. The first step is to establish a baseline. This is going to differ according to what you want to change. Such as; how much time you watch TV, how many cigarettes you smoke each day, how many drinks you consume when out with friends. Then choose how much you're going to give up each week. If you're a smoker and you typically smoke a whole pack a day; then the first week or two you go to 15. Then the next two weeks you go down to 10, and so on until you stop smoking.

7. Don't focus on what you don't want

Most everybody that makes a goal will make this mistake. They will say, I'm not going to do this, or I'm not going to that. Setting a goal like that is setting you up for failure. Instead, decide what you are going to do. It's similar to the bait and switch. If you know you like to snack when working; instead of saying you're not going to snack, say you are going to snack on vegetables. Then all you have to do is switch your chips out for carrots.

8. Do it in honor of yourself

Research shows that people that try to break habits out of frustration or guilt will ultimately fail. People that respect themselves and are happy with who they are will be more successful. Work to change your bad habit from a position of personal strength and confidence.

9. Make a declaration

Social media has become a big part of most everybody's day. Use this to your advantage. Announce on social media the change you are going to make if you feel comfortable doing so. Then keep them updated as you progress. Chances are you will have friends that will congratulate you, and that will make you feel good about what you are doing. This one, of course, isn't for everybody. Some habits that you are trying to break may not be something you want to share with the whole world. Some habits are very personal, so if you don't feel comfortable sharing it with a large group of people, then you don't have to. Keep in mind though having somebody to talk to can help you along the way.

10. Be prepared to forgive yourself

There will be slip-ups. We are only human beings, and we learn from out slip ups. When you slip up, forgive yourself. Wake up the next day ready to beat your habit. Don't go at it with an all or nothing attitude.

There are no scorecards in life. The slip up happened, learn from it, and move on. If you are serious about beating this habit, you won't throw your hands up in defeat after a few lapses.

Classical Conditioning

Classical conditioning is a psychological learning process that occurs when two stimuli are repeatedly paired; a response that is at first elicited by the second stimulus is eventually elicited by the first stimulus alone. An example of this is Pavlov's dog.

Pavlov trained his dog to associate the thrill of being fed with the sound of a bell. He would ring a bell every time he gave the dogs their food. After several repeats of this the dog associated the sound of the bell with receiving food. The dogs would then begin to salivate every time they heard the bell.

This theory doesn't just apply to salivating dogs. Over the years it has formed an important rationale for the development, maintenance, and a relapse of bad habits.

Habits work much in the same way as Pavlov's dogs did. For a smoker, just the site of a pack of cigarettes will elicit a dopamine response causing them to have the urge to smoke. This isn't restricted to smokers either. The same dopamine response happens in alcoholics, overeaters, and so on.

This can be used in reverse, to break a habit. The bell was the trigger for the dogs to start salivating because they knew the food was coming. Just like if a smoker always lights up when they get in the car. The car is the trigger for the smoker to want to smoke. If you start ringing the bell for the dog but don't give them food they will eventually learn that the bell no longer means food. If you stop lighting up every time you get in the car eventually you won't have that trigger anymore.

This is definitely one of the more complicated and harder ways of breaking a habit, but it will work. All the rest have ways of distracting your brain, making it easier to change.

Procrastination

Everybody has been faced with procrastination at some point. It can also be detrimental in your ability to break a habit. But just like breaking a habit, you can overcome procrastination.

In a nutshell, procrastination is when you continually put off doing something. The first step, like with most things, is **realizing you are procrastinating**. If you're honest with yourself, then you know when you are procrastinating, but if you're not sure here are some ways to know;

- Waiting for the right mood, or day to start something
- Doing unimportant tasks to avoid what you need to be doing
- Sitting down to start working, then immediately going to do something else

Once you've realized you are procrastinating, then you can move onto the next step.

Figure out why you are procrastinating. It could be either you or the task. You might find the task unpleasant. Which, since you're changing a habit, you probably will find the task unpleasant. You could also be disorganized or overwhelmed. An important part of the habit breaking process is being organized and knowing what you are doing. Another reason could be that your heart is not into it. You don't have a good enough reason to change this habit.

Lastly, **adopt anti-procrastination strategies**. Procrastination itself is a habit. As you've learned, the only way of getting rid of a habit is persistently not doing the habit. The same tricks you have or will learn about breaking a habit will work to keep you from procrastination. Set up a reward system. Have somebody check in with you. Anything that will keep you accountable in some way, shape, or form.

Be Prepared

Unfortunately, a fact of the world is there will be people that want to sabotage you and your goals. It's not bad enough that you will have self-Sabotaging moments, but you will have to handle other people trying to do the same thing. You have to be prepared to ignore them. They may or may not know what they're doing. Their words can be poison to your success. The moment you start taking their words of "advice" will be your first steps towards failure. Having a plan to handle naysayers is just as important to know what you'll do when you have urges. Make sure you know what to say or do when negative comments arise.

CHAPTER FIVE

A NEW YEAR'S PROBLEM

What's something you get asked every New Year? What's your New Year's resolution? For the first few weeks of the year, every person you see will ask you the same thing. It's expected of everybody to make a New Year's resolution, yet they don't work for people. At least not the way people use them. There's a saying that the definition of insanity is doing the same over and over and again expecting a different result. Then why do people continue to try to make and keep a resolution? People think that resolutions will help them to break some of their bad habits. First, let's look at why a resolution does not work.

1. You're setting the wrong goals.

The most common resolution is to lose weight or get in shape. You wake up the first of January, hop out of bed and say, "I'm going lose 50 pounds this year." By the 15th of January, when you're supposed to be at the gym, you're watching reruns of "The Big Bang Theory" while eating a pint of rocky road. You did nothing wrong. Keeping goals takes more thought than just stating them. These types of goals have little to no leeway. When something happens, and you fail, you will be less likely to make more in the future.

2. Your resolution rarely has to do with the real problem.

You decide to run out and get that gym membership on January first. Good luck fighting the crowd. The gym is going to be packed with everybody else just like you. Once you're in there, you start comparing yourself to everybody. It will definitely help you work through deep-seated psychological issues with inadequacy, rejection, competitiveness and insecurity, but it won't help you solve the real problem. If your goal is to be healthier, then the gym might help, but if you have a problem overeating then it's not going to help. More than likely you're still coming home and eating all the calories you burned off earlier.

3. You set too many.

When making a New Year's resolution a lot of people will think, "While I'm changing this I'll go ahead a change this." Their list of resolutions ends up looking like this;

- Be a better person
- Lose weight
- Sleep more
- Learn a new language
- Drink less

And so on. I get stressed just looking at the list. Our body, as it is, is in homeostasis. It's happy and doesn't want to be changed. The brain has only a finite amount of willpower, and if you start trying to change too many things at once, the brain becomes overwhelmed. The first two weeks of keeping your 10 resolutions may go well, but then your brain starts to smoke and eventually just stops. Then you fall back into old habits.

4. They're too vague.

Let's look at the list above again.

- Be a better person
- Lose weight
- Sleep more
- Learn a new language
- Drink less

They all have something in common. They're about as clear as muddy water. There is no definite way to know if you passed or failed. It's like you teacher gave you an okay on your report card instead of an A or B.

- I want to learn a new language- Great, but what language? Are you trying to learn all languages or a specific one? How are you going to learn your new language? You have no definite plan on how to learn that mysterious new language.

- I want to lose weight- Alright, but how much? Are you overweight and you want to get to a healthier BMI? Do you just want to lose an extra five pounds to fit back into that old dress? You approach those options in very different ways. You have to know how much and why you want to lose weight.

- I want to be a better person- That's admirable, but how? How do you want to be a better person? Do you have a bad temper? Do you use your phone too much? In what way to you want to change? It's great you want to be a better person, but you have to know what aspect of you that you need to change to achieve that goal.

With this new information as to why New Year's resolutions have a tendency to fail, we can now discover how to make them work. No need to swear them off, instead learn how to make them so that you will actually keep them.

1. Be the person you want to be.

The key to keeping any goal is to imagine that you have already achieved your goal. Don't just say, "I'm going to lose weight," or, "I'm going to stop smoking." Be that person. Visualize you eating healthier and working out regularly. Everybody knows the saying "fake it till you make it," this is the same concept. The more you believe on the inside you are already there, the more it will show on the outside.

2. Make them simple.

In fact make them so stupid simple that completing one seems too easy. Remember the acronym KISS, keep it simple stupid. The simpler the goal is, the easier it is to tell that you have accomplished something.

- If you want to drink less hold yourself to drinking one less drink each day, or each week. Then the next week cut out another drink. Continue doing just that, each week, until you reach your overall goal. You'll know you're achieving your goal when you drink less this week than you did the last.

- If you want to sleep more, start setting the alarm to go to bed. If you typically go to bed at midnight, set the alarm on your phone to go off at 10:30 telling you to get ready for bed. That way you will be in bed by eleven. You'll start waking up more refreshed, and you will quickly see that you're achieving your goals.

- If you want to lose weight set your goal to eat more fruits and vegetables each week. Instead of have French fries with your burger have carrot sticks. Start switching out the high-fat sides with whole veggies. You will start seeing a significant change, and you will know you're achieving your goals.

3. Make yourself more accountable.

When people set a resolution, there's nothing that happens to them if they fail, besides the fact that they don't achieve their goal. Instead of having an easy way out, make it painful to not succeed. Dietbet.com is a website that will help you do just that. They have helped over 150,000 people achieve their weight loss goals. The way it works is you choose one of their plans, which you have to pay for. If you achieve your goal, you will win a part of the pot, the money you put in plus some. If you don't achieve your goal, you get nothing. Of course, you don't need their website to do the same thing. If your goal is to quit smoking tell everybody that if you smoke a cigarette, you will pay x amount of dollars to an acquaintance/co-worker/charity that you don't like. Not only are you giving to something or someone you don't like, but you are also spending money that you could use for something you want or need.

4. Keep the number down.

You probably have a million things you want to change, but you have to narrow down your resolution. As I mentioned before your brain only has a finite amount of change willpower. If you deplete it, then you won't achieve anything. Instead make one very simple goal, which is easy to track, and achieve that first. Once you have achieved that goal, and are confident you created a new habit, then start working on another goal.

New Year's resolutions can either help you or hurt you in your habit breaking goal. You have to be extremely careful in the execution. They can be a good way to help you achieve your goals.

CHAPTER SIX

HABIT FORMING

Bad habits. Now we're going to move into a different direction. It's easier, when trying to break a bad habit, to transform it into a good habit. Not only are you eliminating something wrong, you're also forming something good. It's a win-win. Aristotle said, "We are what we repeatedly do. Excellence then is not an act, but a habit." When you were a child learning how to tie your shoes, you had to repeatedly practice over and over again before you learned how. Now you tie your shoes without even thinking. The same goes for forming a new healthy habit.

There are a lot of programs out there that say if you do something for 21 days it will be stuck in your brain. That's true to an extent. Chances are if you have successfully done your goal for 21 days in a row; you will continue to do it. But like all things, it doesn't necessarily work for everybody or every goal. Fulfilling your goal for 21 days is a huge step in the right direction as long as you remember that you still have to actively work to maintain it.

The Three R's

I spoke earlier about the three step structure of forming a habit. You can develop a new habit using that same knowledge. The three R's are; reminder, routine, reward. 'Reminder' is the trigger for your habit. Routine is the habit itself. 'Reward' is the positive thing that makes your brain want to continue to repeat the habit.

Step one is to set a reminder for your new habit. You definitely do need motivation to start a new habit, but motivation isn't enough. And it's definitely not the only way. You have to remember to do your new habit. There are several ways to remind yourself to do something. It could simply be putting your workout clothes someplace where you will see them as soon as you wake up. Set the alarm on your phone telling you to eat a healthy lunch. No matter what it is that you want to start doing, you have to remember to do it.

Picking the right reminder is key, though. The best way I know to figure out when to set a reminder is to make a couple of lists. On the first list write down everything you do every day without fail. For example; brushing your teeth, eating breakfast, going to work, turn off lights, go to bed, and so on. Those are all good things you already do that can remind you to perform your new habit. Such as, after I eat breakfast, I'll go for a walk.

On the second list write down everything that happens to you every day. For example; you stop at a stop sign, you hear your favorite song, a commercial comes on, and you get a text. With both of this list you have a wide array of things that you already respond to that you can use as a reminder. If you want to start moving more, every time you hear your favorite song, dance to it. Don't do this if you're driving, though.

Step two is to create a habit that is super easy to start. There are lots of shows on TV showing people shedding lots of weight in a short amount of time. Or you see the runners or swimmers at the Olympics. It makes you want to achieve the same thing. Everybody has those moments where you think you can be just like them. The enthusiasm is great, but it's important to know that lasting changes are a product of habit. Remember, in the words of Leo Babauta, "Make it so easy that you can't say no." At first, performance doesn't matter. The only thing that matters is you strive to do something. Don't worry about how long you run, or how many veggies you eat, it just matters that you are running or eating vegetables. First, decide what you want your new habit to be. Then ask yourself, "How can I make this so easy that I can't say no?"

Step three is to create a reward. You have to celebrate. Celebration is an important part of life. You want to continue to do something that makes you feel good. Since you have to repeat an action for it to become a habit you have to find a way to reward yourself for doing it. If your goal is to exercise, then every time you finish a work out tell yourself, "Good job," or, "Today was a great day." You can also choose to say "Victory" or "Success" every time you practice the new habit. Give yourself credit no matter how big or small the success was.

Step by Step

That's an easy way to start adopting a new healthy habit. Some habits are going to be harder than others to adopt. Here are few other tips to help adopt a new habit.

Make the habit daily. New habits that you only do every few days are harder to adopt. If you want to start exercising, make sure you exercise once a day for the first 30 days. After the first 30 days, you can step down to three or four times a week.

Write down your goal. When you write out, with pen and paper, what you want your goal to be, it will make it seem more important. It makes your idea more real when you write it down.

Make it so you can't lose. Tell yourself you're running an experiment. You're running an experiment for 30 days by doing this new habit. Experiments can't fail. It makes it seem a lot less stressful. Nothing matters until after the first 30 days, and by that time you have adopted your new habit.

A big downfall of people adopting a new habit is that they doubt there self. When you first start working out you may have the thought, "I can't do this as well as they can." Whenever that thought pops into your head add, "But if I continue to work out I will get better at it." You can use this technique with anything.

Know what could happen. Be sure you know all the consequences of not starting your new habit, and know the impact of starting your new habit. Suppose your goal is eating healthier. If you don't start eating healthier, you could start gaining weight and develop health problems. If you do start eating healthier, you will lose weight and have more energy during the day.

Do it for yourself. Don't bog yourself down with the thoughts of what you should do. Instead, focus on what you want to do. You're making these changes for yourself and not for anybody else. Work towards things that motivate you and make your life better. Don't think you have to live your life like everybody around you does.

Switch Bad for Good

One of the best ways to break a bad habit is to switch it out for a good one. It helps to trick your brain and contributes to reduce cravings.

- As always, you have to first identify your triggers. You cannot break bad habits until you figure out what triggers them.
- For every trigger identify a good habit that you could do instead. Instead of smoking when you wake up, what are you

going to do? Good habits could be; exercise, meditation, decluttering, organizing, and more.

- For, at least a month, be consistent with those triggers. Every time a trigger comes up act on the good habit you decided to do. The more consistent you are, the more the new habit will become ingrained, and the less you will think of the bad habit.

- Avoid severe trigger situations. You can't always switch out all triggers for new habits. As mentioned before, you might want to skip going out with friends after work for a little while. At least until you get a handle on controlling your urges.

- Discover ways to fight the strong urges. Even though the goal is to switch out the bad habit for a good habit, you will still get the urge to do the bad habit. You will likely need a backup plan when fighting urges.

- Find supportive help. Have somebody you can talk to if things get really rough. Some bad habits are tougher to break than others, and you will go through some tough times, so having somebody you can talk to will help you work through the tough times.

- Stay positive. There will be times when negative thoughts pop into your head. You will have self-sabotaging moments. But the key is to stay positive. When negative thoughts come up, remind yourself why you're doing this. Remind yourself that you're changing yourself for the better.

CHAPTER SEVEN

BE SUPPORTIVE

The human mind has the amazing ability to be able to talk you out of doing what you know is right. It can come up with crazy reasons why you shouldn't do something that you know you need to do. You want to work out, "Why? It will make you sweaty." You want to quit smoking, "You'll feel more stress if you do." You want to go to be earlier, "But then you'll miss Jimmy Kimmel." See what I mean. You have to find a way to tell your brain to shut up, and an accountability partner will help you do just that.

Growing up you probably had friends that you would vent to, and they would help you feel better about a situation. An accountability partner works much in the same way.

It will probably feel foreign or uncomfortable the first time. That's a good thing. The uncomfortable feeling is your brain resisting the change. Embrace those feelings. It will be worth it once you work through them.

The role of an accountability partner is to keep you accountable. They help as an outside force to tell your brain to shut up. Their only purpose is to keep you on track. They are there for you when you feel like straying from your path. They're there for you when you wake up in the middle of the night wanting a cupcake. Or when you are extremely stressed out, and you want a cigarette.

Your partner can be anybody that you resonate with. There is no need to pay a professional. They could be a family member, co-worker, friend, or somebody else that is trying to achieve the same goal. Find someone that you connect with and trust to hold you accountable. Be completely open about your goal. What you want to achieve and when you want to achieve it. They are there to be your cheerleader and to hold you to your commitment. Here are some things to look for in choosing your accountability partner:

1. They're reliable. They are easily reached whenever wherever.

2. They want to be your partner. You can’t make somebody help you, so make sure they actually want to.

3. Make sure they can relate to you in some way. You don't want to pick someone that has never tried to lose weight to help you lose weight. They won't understand what you're going through.
4. You feel comfortable being honest and open with them, and they are comfortable giving you honest feedback.

Now that you know how to pick your accountability partner, let's talk about the benefits they will provide you. One of the biggest benefits to having an accountability partner is they will accelerate your performance. When you connect with someone one-on-one, you are able to work through the problems of your plan with them. You'll be able to make a sure fire plan to achieve your goals.

Your partner will help you measure your achievements. A good partner will help you to set milestones to reach along the way. It will be easier for you to keep track of your success, and keep you from becoming discouraged. Their outside eyes will see your success more easily than you will be able to.

They will help to validate your thoughts and ideas. Having someone to bounce your ideas off of, besides yourself, will help you to make decisions. They can give you honest outside information. They will help to silence your inner critic.

They help to keep you engaged. Things will come up that will try to distract you from your goals, and you will have someone there to help you stay the path. When you're bored, they will be there for you to talk to. Just knowing that you have somebody there for you will help you to keep your eye on the prize.

Ultimately they will hold you responsible. They are there behind you, pushing you towards your goals. They keep you from getting distracted and hold you accountable. Having a weekly check in with someone, and knowing you have to tell them what you have done this week to achieve your goal, will make you more likely to stay proactive. They keep you from making excuses, and, instead, make deliberate actions towards your end goal.

This isn't to say that you can't achieve your goals by yourself. There are people out there that can, but it takes a lot more willpower. Having a support system will make all the difference in the world.

CHAPTER EIGHT

BOOST YOUR POWER

And that's willpower. Willpower is probably one of the last things you need to work on though. If you don't know what you're trying to change, or why you're doing it, then willpower isn't going to help. You could have great willpower, but without a purpose it's going to fall flat. It's like building a house. You can have all the wood you need, but if you don't have the nails, it's not going to stay together. Once you have your plan in place, then you can move onto willpower.

Willpower and self-control are imperative building blocks for a happy and prosperous life. Some of the most persuasive evidence comes from these two studies.

The first is the marshmallow experiment. Psychologist Walter Mischel started the experiment in the 1960s. He would offer four-year-olds a choice of a marshmallow now or two marshmallows if they could wait 15 minutes. He and his associates then tracked those students as they grew up. They found that the children who were willing to wait 15 minutes for the marshmallows achieved greater academic success, better health, and a less likely chance of divorce.

In the second study, 1,000 children were studied from birth to 32. Researchers found that the children's self-control could predict the future of their health, substance dependence, criminal offenses, and personal finances. It was even true when they eliminated factors such as intelligence and social class.

Use it or lose it

Everybody knows these two factors about muscles:

- Muscles get stronger when exercised
- Muscles can be overworked, which leaves them weak until they have time to rest

But here are some interesting things you may not know.

- In a study, some participants were told not to think about a white bear. Thought-suppression takes a good deal of self-control, especially when told not to think about something. After that, they were told to limit their intake of beer during a taste test because there would be a driving test later. The thought-suppression participants drank more than the non-thought-suppression participants.

- In another study, participants that were asked to suppress their emotions during an upsetting movie gave up sooner during a physical stamina test than those who were freely allowed to express their emotions.

- In a third study, women watched a documentary while seated near a candy bowl. In some, the candy bowl was right next to the woman, in others the candy bowl was across the room from them. Later, they were given hard puzzles to solve. Those that had been seated close to the candy bowl gave up sooner than those who weren't.

In each of these studies, the people that were forced to overuse their willpower or self-control could not fully finish subsequent tasks. Their willpower had been depleted. Now let's look at some ways to strengthen your willpower.

1. Don't keep your willpower depleted

If you have plans to help your friend move heavy pieces of furniture, you're not going to spend 30 minutes before lifting weights. You know your energy will be depleted before you help your friend. The same goes for your willpower. Exercising self-control is an excellent way to build willpower, never giving yourself a break is a good way to deplete it.

2. Meditation

Meditation seems to come up a lot when looking for ways to change habits. It is a great way to strengthen your ability to control your thoughts. But what is meditation? Meditation is simply the practice of bringing your thoughts to the present moment. 47% of lives are spent either thinking about the past, or what has to be done in the future. Leaving us with very little time to think about what we are doing at this present moment. Our brains are very undisciplined. They like to wander. With 10 minutes of meditation each day it will help strengthen your mind and help keep it from wandering. Studies have shown after just 2 to 3 days of 10-minute meditation your brain will be able to focus better, you will have more energy and a lot less stress.

3. Use your imagination

Imagination is an amazing way to improve willpower. The body can respond the same way to an imaginary scenario as the real one. If you imagine laying on a beach, listening to the waves crash, your body will respond by relaxing. On the other hand, if you think about going to work and having a meeting with your boss, your body will tense in response. Dieters are in a constant state of depletion. As a result, they feel everything more intensely. Imagination is able to help control these irritations

In a study, participants were asked to watch a movie with a bowl of chocolate placed nearby. One group was told to imagine they had decided to eat as much as they want. The second group was told to imagine they had eaten none. The third group was told to imagine they had decided to eat the chocolate later. The first group ate more than the other two. Then when given the opportunity to eat later, those that had imagined they would eat later, ate less than the others. They even reported a lesser desire to consume the candy.

4. Use your opposite hand

Researchers have conducted studies that tested corrective actions. One they found that worked particularly well was to use your opposite hand. Your brain is wired to use your dominant hand so it will take willpower to use the non-dominate hand. To practice this, choose a time during the day to use your non-dominate hand. I would suggest doing no more than an hour at a time. More than an hour may deplete your willpower

5. Distract yourself

It's even possible to use your imagination to distract yourself from unwanted thoughts. Just like in the study mentioned earlier about the white bear. When you tell yourself not to think about something, it's going to continually pop back into your head. Train yourself to think about something else. If you don't want to think about that white bear, or cigarettes, or candy, flip your thoughts to something else. Instead of a white bear, think of a black bear. Instead of cigarettes, think of chewing gum. Instead of candy, think of fruit. That puts you in complete control of your thoughts

6. Control your stress

I have mentioned stress several times throughout this book. Stress is the main culprit of many problems. When you become stressed, you'll tend to fall back into old habits. Most of the time you won't even realize it because your body goes into autopilot. When you're stressed, your body releases stress hormones, mainly cortisol.

Cortisol increases your cravings for carbohydrates. Carbs will lower your cortisol levels. Which is probably perhaps why you turn to your friends Ben and Jerry. Alcohol is also a depressant that reduces your cortisol levels. Both of those options hold some negative side effect and aren't helping you to kick those bad habits.

Fortunately, we know these things so you can have control over what you do. The stress response is the same as the fight or flight response, so anything that counterattacks that response will do. Start responding to those stressors by listening to calming music, visualizing calming scenes, or moderate exercise. Whatever works for you. Researchers also say viewing funny videos can help counteract willpower depletion.

The more you practice these habits, the more likely they will be there to help you when major stressors arise.

7. A step at a time

Most of the time people give up on goals, not because of the lack of willpower, but because of feeling overwhelmed in what they are trying to accomplish. I have mentioned something similar to this before. Break your goals down into manageable pieces. That way you can see each step you take instead of trying to consume the whole thing. This also keeps you from depleting your willpower, keeping you recharged and ready to continue working at all times.

8. Be yourself

It takes a lot of effort to suppress you typical behaviors, personality, and preferences. Not surprisingly, it also depletes willpower. Psychologist Mark Muraven found that people who exert self-control to make others happy were more easily depleted than individuals who held true to their own goals and happiness. People pleasures may find they are at a disadvantage when it comes to willpower as opposed to those who are secure and comfortable with their self.

9. Change your speech

In another correction study, researchers conducted to modify the subject's natural speech. This would include resisting the urge to say a cuss word, or simply change from saying "hey" to "hello." It takes willpower to make the conscious effort to change one's speech, especially when we typically speak out of instinct. It doesn't matter what you do to change your speech, as long as you make a conscious effort to switch things up. Just like using your opposite hand, choose a chunk of your day where you will change the way you speak. You also need to decide what it is that you are going to change. You might choose to stop swearing, or to stop saying slang words like "ain't." Remember to only practice this for about an hour at a time, or you may deplete your willpower. After only two weeks you will see an increase in your willpower.

10. Keep temptations at bay

With most habits, you have a weakness for what you like to consume. If you drink too much keep alcohol out of your house. If you smoke, get rid of all your cigarettes. If you snack a lot, either get rid of the junk food or put it out of sight. There will be times when you see your weakness, and you will need to make a plan for that moment. Decide how you are going to handle it. If your weakness is junk food and you have children, chances are junk food is going to enter your house at some point. No matter where the kids got the food, grandma, trick or treating, school, work out a plan where you don't constantly see it. Work with your spouse or significant other. Have them take all the junk food and put it where you don't know where it is. If the kids want some, they have to ask the other parent, not you. And you have to promise that you won't beg and plead to know where it is. That takes a little willpower in itself, but a lot less than trying to keep from eating the junk food that you see.

Willpower is just like any other muscle in your body. With the right practice, it can be strengthened. I have just given you 10 ways to increase your willpower and self-control, but don't try to do all 10 at once. You'll just end up driving yourself crazy. Think of training your willpower just like you would prepare for a race. On your first day of training, you're not going to run the full 26 miles. Not unless you're already an Olympic runner. Instead, you will increase the amount you run every day. Choose one of these to start using on a daily basis. Once you feel that's not working for you anymore, pick a different one. Before you know it, you will be more mentally strong.

CHAPTER NINE

MEDITATIVE STATE

Mediation has proved to be very helpful in most aspects of life. It has shown up numerous times already in this book. Since it seems to be so useful, I figured I would dedicate a whole chapter to it. We'll take a deeper look into the benefits of meditation and how it will help you break your bad habits. Then I will give you a simple step by step on how to get started meditating for beginners. If you already meditate, then you have a leg up.

Ask anybody that meditates, and they will tell you it's good for you. But in what way? Is that just from years of practice, or is there scientific research out there that proves it's good for you? Here are some general ways that mediation can help:

- Improves willpower
- Improves focus
- Decreases stress
- Improves ability to learn

- Increases energy

There are over 3,000 scientific studies that examine the benefits of meditation. I'm going to summarize some of the findings for you.

- Decreases depression

In Belgium, a study was conducted at five middle schools involving approximately 400 students. Professor Filip Raes concluded that the students that participated in mindfulness meditation reduced indication of anxiety, stress, and depression for up to six months later. At the University of California, a similar study was conducted with formerly depressive patients and concluded that mindfulness meditation reduced ruminative thinking and dysfunctional beliefs.

- Reduces panic disorder

The American Journal of Psychiatry published a study where 22 patients diagnosed with panic disorder were submitted to 3 months of meditation and relaxation training. 20 of the 22 participants showed that their panic and anxiety had been reduced significantly, and the changes were maintained at follow-up.

- Increases concentration

Harvard neuroscientists ran an experiment where 16 people took part in an 8-week mindfulness course. They used guided meditation and integration of mindfulness in everyday activities. Sara Lazer, Ph.D., reported at the end, MRI scans showed that gray matter concentration increased in areas of the brain involved in learning, memory, emotion regulation, sense of self, and perspective.

- Increases focus in spite of distraction

Emory University did a study that demonstrated that participants with more mediation experience exhibited increased connectivity within the brain controlling attention. The neural relationships may be involved in the development of cognitive skills.

- Prevents you from falling in a multitasking trap

Multitasking is a dangerous productivity myth that will deplete you of energy and is a source of stress. Switching between tasks is costly to your brain which can cause feelings of distraction and dissatisfaction. In a study conducted by the University of Washington and the University of Arizona, human resources personnel took part in 8 weeks of in either mindfulness meditation or body relaxation techniques. They were given stressful multitasking tests before and after training. Groups that had practice meditation showed lower stress levels and a better recall of the tasks they had done. They also switched between tasks less often, concentrating on one task for a longer amount of time.

- Increases unconscious mind awareness

A study done by the University of Sussex found that people who practiced mindfulness meditation experienced a longer paused between unconscious impulses and action. They were also less susceptible to hypnosis.

- Reduces heart diseases and stroke

Cardiovascular disease kills more people in the world than anything else. A study performed in 2012, studied 200 high-risk individuals. They were asked to, either, take part in a health education class promoting better diet and exercise, or take a class on transcendental meditation. During the next five years, they found that those who took the meditation class decreased their overall risk of heart disease, stroke, and death by 48%.

- Increases compassion and decreases worry

After 9 weeks of compassion cultivation training, participants showed significant improvement in all three domains of compassion (compassion for others, receiving compassion, and self-compassion).

- Decreases emotional eating

Scientists have found that transcendental meditation decreases the likelihood of emotional eating, which helps to prevent obesity.

There is a lot more scientific information out there that proves meditation can help with all aspects of life. It's no wonder that it shows up a lot in contributing to quit bad habits.

Simple meditation practice

If you've never meditated before, I would suggest doing a guided meditation. A quick search on the internet will turn up several apps and downloads for guided meditation. Some free choices are Omvana, Headspace, Calm, Smiling Mind, and Take a Break.

If you want to meditate on your own here is a simple meditation practice designed by Headspace App founder, Andy Puddicombe:

1. Find a quiet room where you can sit comfortably upright with no distraction.

2. Set a 10-minute timer, and get comfortable in your chair.

3. Find something in your line of vision to focus on for 6 deep breaths. With each exhale, allow your body to soften as you become more relaxed. On the 6th exhale, close your eyes.

4. Focus your attention on the points of contact between your body and the chair and floor. Notice the sensation of your arms, back, and bottom on the chair, and your feet on the floor.

5. Then become aware of your surroundings. Notice all the sounds and smells around you. Anything that you can sense without your sight.

6. Then focus on your breath. Notice how your chest expands when you breathe in and how it contracts when you exhale.

7. Once you're comfortable with the rhythm of your breathing, begin to count. 1 on the inhale, 2 on the exhale, all the way up to 10. This will keep your mind focused on your breath and keep it from wandering.

8. When you make it to 10, start back over at 1. Do not count 11, 12, 13, etc.

9. While you breathe, allow your thoughts to come and go. You can't stop yourself from thinking. What you want to do is avoid lingering on one thought. The moment you realize your mind has wandered, bring it back to your breaths.

10. Continue until your timer goes off.

The first time you do this, it will probably seem awkward and weird. It's just like adopting a new habit. The more you do it, the less uncomfortable it becomes, and the easier it will be to do.

Here are some other, more advanced, mediation options:

- Candle starting

If you have problems focusing, you can light a candle and stare at it. Make sure the candle is at eye level. If you find your mind wandering, return your focus to what the flame is doing. Another level up is to stare at the candle without blinking. It will eventually make you cry which refreshes your eyes.

- Mantra

The repetition of words helps you to find calm and focus. You can find different mantras online, or you can make up your own. It doesn't matter what you say as long as it resonates with you, and you're happy with it.

- Visualization

Another fun and easy way to meditate is to visualize an idyllic being or setting in your mind. You can make it whatever you want. Embellishing it as much or as little as you need.

- Become the Observer

Become the observer of your mind. Close your eyes and focus on the spot, about an inch, above the spot between your eyebrows, third eye chakra. Begin to focus on what you mind and body is feeling, thinking and doing.

You should now be able to use meditation to help you break your bad habits, and, in the process, start a new good, habit.

I'm sure you are dying to start working on getting rid of that bad habit that's been bothering you, so I'll wrap this up. Remember to keep this simple. Don't overwhelm yourself with too many goals, or trying too many of these techniques at once. Be prepared to fail and meet naysayers, they are inevitable, but you don't have to let them control you. If nothing else, please remember you deserve to live the best life possible.

PART V

Chapter 1: Identifying the Mediterranean Diet

We know that certain diets are associated with better health—this is a simple fact of life. We've seen that entire groups of people live longer based on where they live, and to some degree, a good deal of that has to come from somewhere—it has to come from something like diet or environment. In this case, the diet of the people living in the Mediterranean has been found to be incredibly healthy for people—it has been shown that people who are able to enjoy this diet, who are able to eat fresh food by the sea and enjoy the benefits that it has, are able to be far healthier than those who don't have it. That is great for them—but what is their secret?

It turns out, it's all in the lifestyle. The Mediterranean lifestyle, food, and all, is incredibly healthy for you. Studies have shown that people living in Mediterranean countries such as Greece and Italy have been found to have far less risk of death from coronary disease. Their secret is in the diet. Their diet has been shown to reduce the risk of cardiovascular disease, meaning that it is incredibly healthy, beneficial, and something that the vast majority of people in the world could definitely benefit from.

The Mediterranean diet is recommended by doctors and the World Health Organization as being not only healthy but also sustainable, meaning that it is something that is highly recommended, even by the experts. If you've found that you've struggled with weight loss, heart disease, managing your blood pressure, or anything similar to those problems, then the Mediterranean diet is for you.

When you follow this diet, you are able to bring health back to your life and enjoy the foods while doing so. It's perfect if you want to be able to enjoy your diet without having to worry about the impacts that it will have on you.

Defining the Mediterranean Lifestyle

The Mediterranean diet is quite simple. It involves eating traditional foods based on one's location. Typically, in the Mediterranean, that is a diet that is rich in veggies, fruits, whole grains, beans, and features olive oil as the fat of choice. Typically, it involves elements beyond just eating as well. While it is important to have healthy food, it is equally important to recognize that the diet encompasses the lifestyle as well. In particular, you can expect to see a few other rules come into play.

In particular, the Mediterranean diet is unique in the sense that it encourages a glass of red wine every now and then. In fact, the diet is associated with moderate drinking, enjoying red wine several times per week, always responsibly, and in contexts that will be beneficial to the drinker. If you want to be able to enjoy the Mediterranean diet and you are pregnant, or against drinking, you can do that, too—but traditionally, the red wine is included and even encouraged in moderation thanks to the antioxidants within it.

Additionally, on the Mediterranean diet, it is common to share meals with friends and family. This is essential—eating is more than just filling the body, it is nurturing the mind and relationships as well. This also comes with the added benefit of also being able to slow down eating—when you are eating the foods on this diet, you will discover that ultimately, you eat less when you're busy having a riveting conversation with someone. The fact that you are slowed down with your eating means that you will fill up sooner and realize that you didn't have to actually eat the food that you did. This means that you eat less and are, therefore managing your portions better as a result.

Finally, the Mediterranean diet focuses on physical activity. Traditionally, you would have had to go out to get the foods that you would eat each day, and that would mean that you'd need to get up, fish, garden, farm, or otherwise prepare your food. Eating locally is still a major component of this diet, as is getting up and being active. You need at least 30 minutes of activity, moderate or mild, per day. Even just walking for half an hour is better than nothing!

The Rules of the Mediterranean Diet

To eat the Mediterranean way, there are a few key factors that can guide you. If you know what you are doing, you can eat well without having to sacrifice flavor for health, and that matters immensely. When you look at the Mediterranean diet closely, you see that there are several tips that will help you to recognize what you need to do to stick to your diet.

Eating fruits and veggies

First, make sure that the bulk of your calories come from fruits and vegetables. You should be eating between 7 and 10 servings of fresh fruits and vegetables every single day—meaning that the bulk of your calories will come from there. Try to stick to locally grown foods that are fresh and in-season—they will have the highest nutritional value.

Reach for the whole grains

Yes, pasta is a major part of the diet in the Mediterranean, and you don't have to give that up entirely—but make sure that any grains that you are enjoying are whole-wheat. This allows you to enjoy foods that are high in fiber and are able to be digested differently than when you use refined carbs instead. While the refined carbs may give you instantaneous energy, they are also not nearly as good for you as whole wheat.

Using healthy fats

When it comes to flavoring or cooking your foods, you need to reach for the healthy fats first. This means choosing out foods that are cooked with olive oil instead of butter or dipping food in olive oil instead of butter. Olive oil, despite being a fat, has not been found to lead to weight gain when used in moderation. It is an incredibly healthy substitute for butter that is loaded up with all sorts of beneficial, heart-healthy antioxidants that will help your cardiovascular system.

Aim for seafood

When it comes to protein, fish, especially fresh fish, is the best choice. Fish should be consumed at least twice per week, and it should be fresh rather than frozen whenever possible. In particular, it is commonly recommended that you reach for salmon or trout, or other fatty fish because the omega-3 fatty acids within them are incredibly healthy for you, and they will serve you well. Even better, if you grill your fish, you have little cleanup.

Reduce red meat

In addition to adding more seafood to your diet, you need to cut out the red meat. The red meats in your diet are no good for you—they have been linked to inflammation that can make it harder for your cardiovascular system.

Enjoy dairy in moderation

When you are on this diet, dairy is not out of the picture entirely. While you should avoid butter, for the most part, it is a good idea for you to enjoy some low-fat Greek yogurt on occasion and add in some cheese to your diet. It is a good thing for you to enjoy these foods to ensure that you have plenty of calcium to keep your body strong.

Spices, not salt

Perhaps one of the most profound differences between most other diets and the Mediterranean diet is the lack of salt. The Mediterranean diet reaches for herbs and spices before adding in salt, meaning that you will be consuming less of it over time. Even better, you will grow to love your new foods without needing salt.

Chapter 2: Savory Mediterranean Meals

Mediterranean Feta Mac and Cheese

Ingredients

- Egg (1, beaten)
- Feta cheese (8 oz., crumbles)
- Macaroni (0.5 lb., whole-wheat)
- Olive oil (3 Tbsp.)
- Salt and pepper to taste
- Sour cream (8 oz.)

Instructions

1. Cook pasta to instructions to create al dente pasta. Drain and place pasta into baking dish. Toss in feta and oil and mix well.
2. Combine your egg and sour cream with salt and pepper. Then mix well and toss over macaroni. Combine and bake at 350F for 30 minutes.

Chickpea Stew

Ingredients

- Bay leaf (1)
- Dry chickpeas (1 c., soaked overnight and peeled)
- Garlic (1 clove, cut in half)
- Lemon to serve
- Olive oil (0.25 c.)
- Onion (1, diced)
- Salt and pepper to taste

Instructions

1. Cover chickpeas in pot with just enough water to cover them and wait to boil. Then rinse and set into clean pot. Toss in all other ingredients but the lemon with just enough water to cover nearly one inch above the beans. Simmer for 2-3 hours and serve with lemons.

Savory Mediterranean Breakfast Muffins

Ingredients

Dry ingredients

- Baking powder (1.5 tsp)
- Baking soda (o.5 tsp)
- Flour (2 c.)
- Salt (0.5 tsp)

Wet ingredients

- Egg (1 large)
- Garlic (1 clove, minced)
- Milk (1 c.)
- Sour cream (0.25 c.)
- Vegetable oil (0.25 c.)

Fillings

- Cheddar cheese (2 c., shredded)
- Feta (2.5 oz., crumbled)
- Green olives (diced, 0.5 c.)
- Green onions (0.5 c., chopped)
- Roasted red peppers (0.5 c., chopped)
- Sun dried tomatoes (diced, 0.5 c.)

Instructions

1. Combine dry ingredients in a bowl. Mix wet ingredients in separate bowl. Combine the two together and mix.
2. Toss in fillings in as few stirs as possible.

3. Place in greased or lined muffin pan, dividing to all 12 recesses.
4. Bake for 25 minutes until golden-brown and crusty at 350F.
5. Cool for 10 minutes and serve warm.

Mediterranean Breakfast Bake

Ingredients

- Artichoke hearts (14-oz. can, drained)
- Bread (6 slices whole-wheat, chopped)
- Eggs (8)
- Feta cheese (0.5 c.)
- Italian sausage (turkey or chicken—1 lb., casings removed)
- Milk (1 c.)
- Olive oil (2 Tbsp., divided)
- Onion (1, chopped)
- Spinach (5 oz.)
- Sun dried tomato (1 c., chopped)

Instructions

1. Warm 1 Tbsp. of your olive oil on moderately high heat. Cook sausage for 8 minutes until it has browned, breaking it up as it cooks. Place it in a dish when it is done.
2. Toss in additional oil, then cook onion until soft, roughly 5 minutes. Toss in spinach until wilting (1 minute).
3. Combine eggs and mix in milk, bread, tomatoes, cheese, artichokes, sausage, and finally, the spinach mix.
4. Place everything in a 2.5 quart baking dish. Let sit for an hour in fridge, or leave overnight.
5. Let casserole sit for 30 minutes after removing from fridge. Then, bake for 45 minutes at 350F until brown. Let rest 10 minutes, then serve.

Mediterranean Pastry Pinwheels

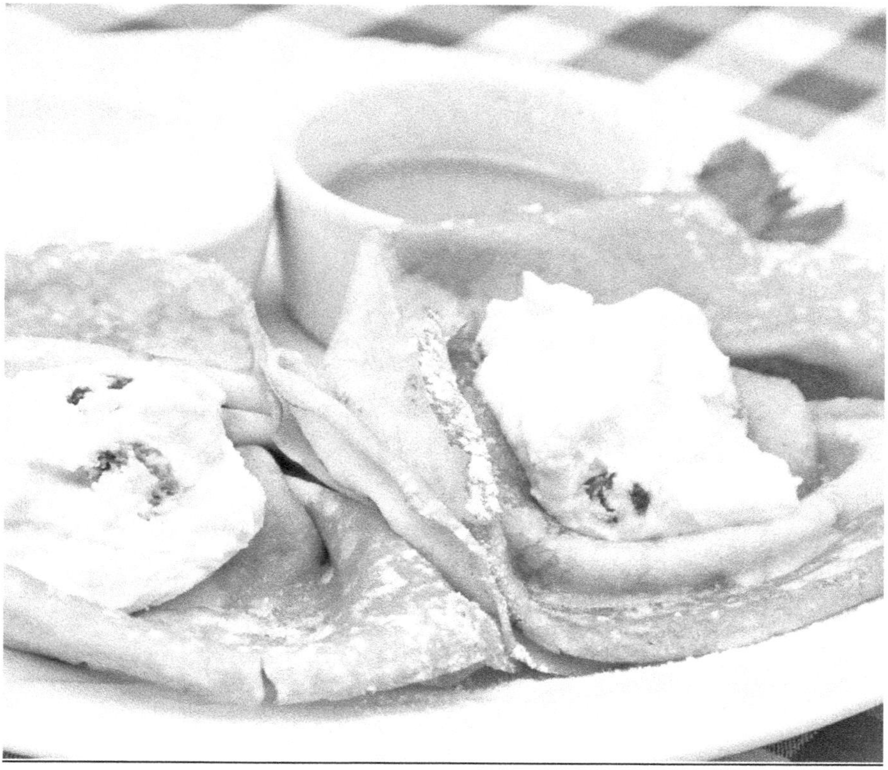

Ingredients

- Cream cheese (8-ounce package, softened)
- Pesto (0.25 c.)
- Provolone cheese (0.75 c.)
- Sun-dried tomatoes (0.5 c., chopped)
- Ripe olives (0.5 c., chopped)

Instructions

1. Unroll pastry and trim it up to create 10-inch square.
2. Mix together your cream cheese and pesto until well-combined. Then, mix in other ingredients until combined. Place mixture in even layer across pastry, up to 0.5-inch of edges. Roll and freeze for 30 minutes.
3. Cut whole roll into 16 pieces.
4. Bake at 400F until golden, roughly 15 minutes. Serve.

Chapter 3: Sweet Treats on the Mediterranean Diet

Greek Yogurt Parfait

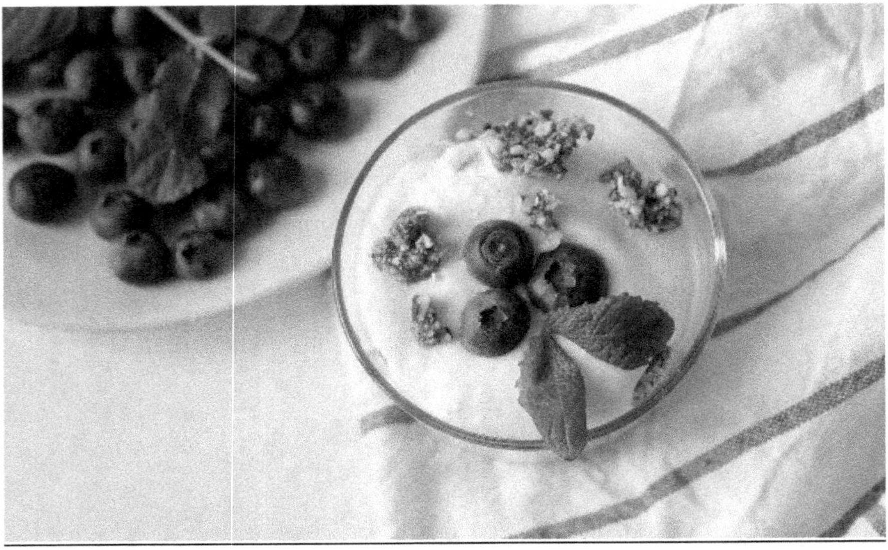

Ingredients

- Almond butter (2 Tbsp.)
- Fresh fruit (1 Tbsp.)
- Greek Yogurt (1 c.)

Instructions

1. Mix together yogurt and 1 Tbsp. of almond butter and put in a bowl. Top with fruit.
2. Warm remaining butter in microwave for 10 minutes, then drizzle atop yogurt. Serve. You can add different toppings to change up the flavor as well.

Overnight Oats

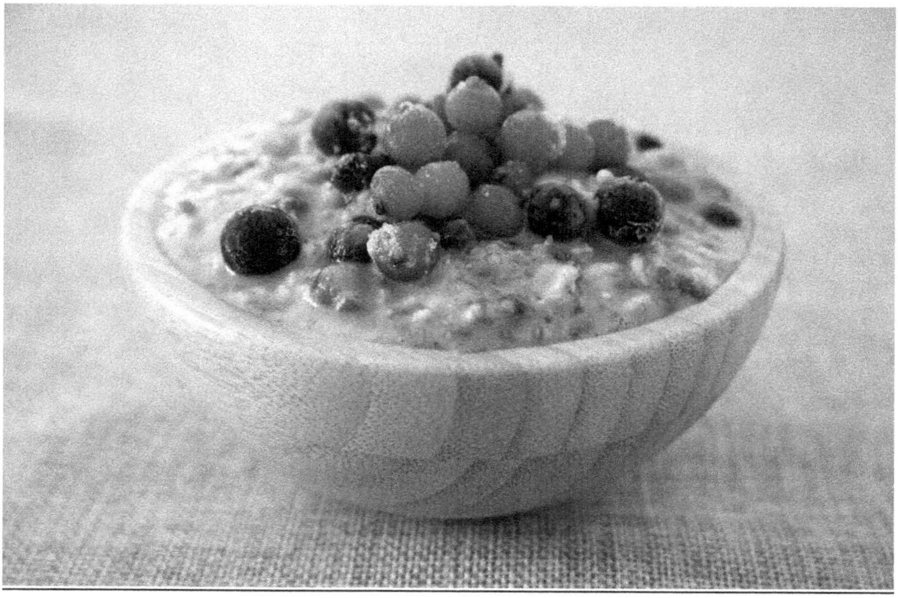

Ingredients

- Chia seeds (1 Tbsp.)
- Greek yogurt (0.25 c.)
- Honey (1 Tbsp.)
- Milk of choice (0.5 c.)
- Old fashioned whole oats (0.5 c.)
- Vanilla extract (0.25 tsp)

Instructions

1. Mix all ingredients into a glass container and leave in fridge for at least 2 hours but preferably overnight. Serve with berries of choice or other desired toppings.

Apple Whipped Yogurt

Ingredients

- Greek yogurt (1 c.)
- Heavy cream (0.5 c.)
- Honey (1 Tbsp.)
- Unsalted butter (2 Tbsp.)
- Apples (2, cored and chopped into small bits)
- Sugar (2 Tbsp.)
- Cinnamon (1/8 tsp)
- Walnut halves (0.25 c., chopped)

Instructions

1. Using a hand mixer, mix together yogurt, honey, and honey until it creates peaks.
2. Heat up your butter in a skillet over a moderate temperature. Cook apples and 1 Tbsp. sugar in pan. Stir and cook for 6-8 minutes until soft. Then, top with the rest of sugar and cinnamon, stirring and cooking an additional 3 minutes. Take it off of the burner and let it rest for 5 minutes.
3. Serve with whipped yogurt in bowl topped with apple, then sprinkle on walnuts.

Chapter 4: Gourmet Meals on the Mediterranean Diet

Garlic-Roasted Salmon and Brussels Sprouts

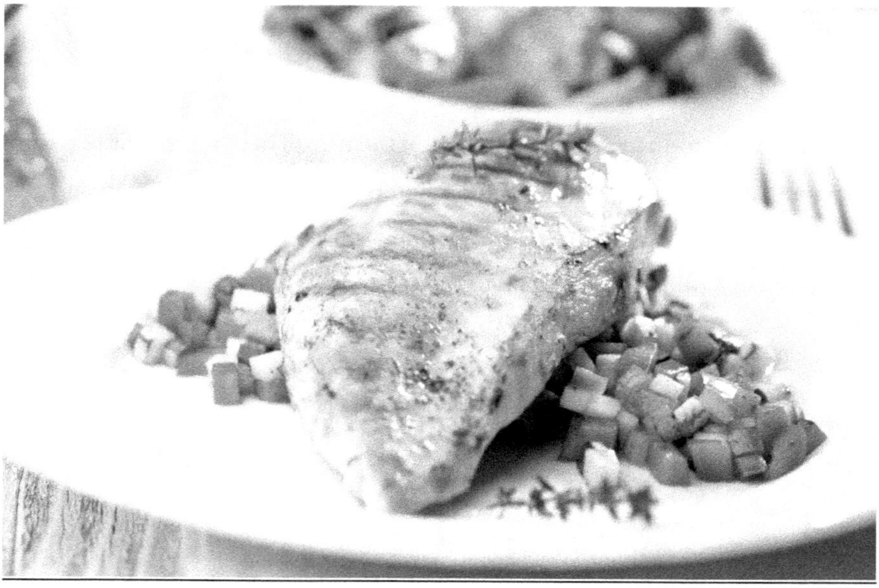

Ingredients

- Brussels sprouts (6 c., trimmed and halved)
- Chardonnay (0.75 c.)
- Garlic cloves (14 large)
- Olive oil (0.25 c.)
- Oregano (2 Tbsp., fresh)
- Pepper (0.75 tsp)
- Salmon fillet (2 lbs., skin-off—cut in 6 pieces)
- Salt (1 tsp)
- Lemon wedges to serve

Instructions

1. Take two cloves of garlic and mince, combining them with oil, 1 Tbsp. of oregano, half of the salt and 1/3 of the pepper. Cut remaining cloves of garlic in halves and toss them with the sprouts. Take 3 Tbsp. of your garlic oil and toss it with the sprouts in roasting pan. Roast for 15 minutes at 450F.
2. Add wine to the remainder of the oil mixture. Then, remove it from the pan, stir veggies, and place salmon atop it all. Pour the wine mix atop it and season with remaining oregano and salt and pepper. Bake 5-10 minutes until salmon is done. Serve alongside the wedged lemon.

Walnut Crusted Salmon with Rosemary

Ingredients

- Dijon mustard (2 tsp)
- Garlic (1 clove, minced)
- Honey (0.5 tsp)
- Kosher salt (0.5 tsp)
- Lemon juice (1 tsp)
- Lemon zest (0.25 tsp.)
- Olive oil (1 tsp)
- Olive oil spray
- Panko (3 Tbsp.)
- Red pepper (0.25 tsp)
- Rosemary (1 tsp, chopped)

- Salmon (1 pound, skin removed)
- Walnuts (3 Tbsp., finely chopped)
- Parsley and lemon to garnish

Instructions

1. Mix together the mustard, lemon zest and juice, honey, salt and red pepper, and rosemary. In a separate dish, combine the panko with oil and walnuts.
2. Spread mustard across salmon and top with panko mixture. Spray fillets with cooking spray.
3. Cook until fish begins to flake at 425F, roughly 8-10 minutes. Serve with lemon and parsley.

Spaghetti and Clams

Ingredients

- Clams (6.5 lbs.)
- Olive oil (6 Tbsp.)
- White wine (0.5 c.)
- Garlic (3 cloves, sliced)
- Chiles (3, small and crumbled)
- Spaghetti (1 lb.)
- Parsley (3 Tbsp., chopped)
- Salt and pepper to personal preference

Instructions

1. Prepare clams, soaking in clean water and brushing to remove all sand.

2. Warm 2 Tbsp. of oil in large pot. Then, toss in 0.25 c. wine, 1 of the cloves of garlic, and 1 chile. Cook half of the plans at high heat with regular shaking until clams are opened. Remove opened clams and their juices to a larger bowl. Repeat process with second half of clams. Discard any that do not open.
3. Prepare pasta according to packaging to create al dente pasta. Reserve 1 c. pasta water.
4. Warm remainder of oil (2 Tbsp.) in pot over moderate heat, tossing in remainder of garlic and chile. Cook until fragrant, then place all clams and their juices into the pot, tossing to coat well. Then, toss in pasta, mixing well to combine. If necessary, add in cooking liquid. Serve and season with salt/pepper to personal preference with parsley atop.

Braised Lamb and Fennel

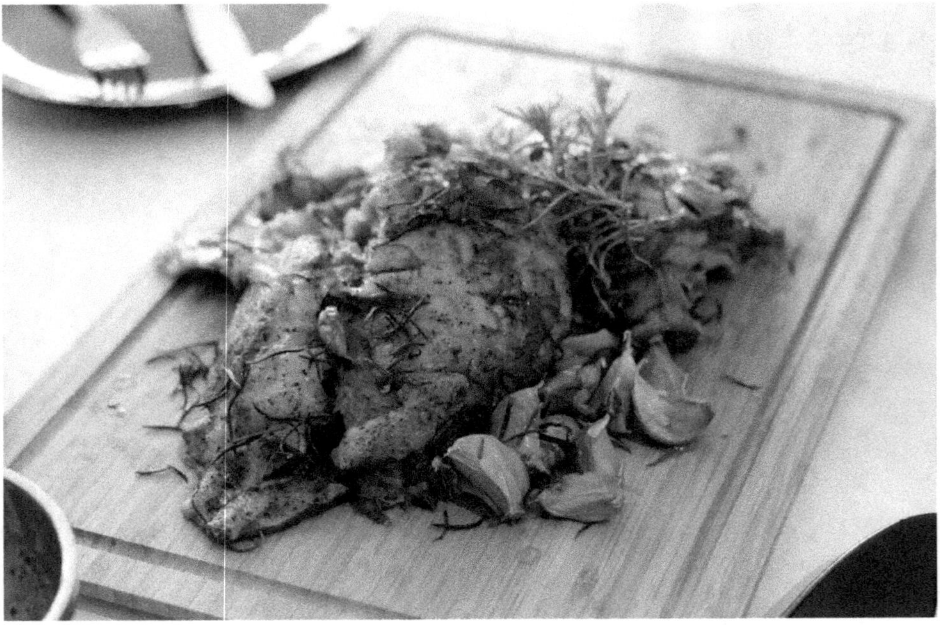

Ingredients

- Bay leaves (2)
- Chicken broth (3 c.)
- Cinnamon stick (1)
- Fennel (1 bulb, chopped)
- Garlic head (chopped in half)
- Lamb shoulder (3 lbs., cut into 8 pieces)
- Olive oil (2 Tbsp.)
- Onion (1, chopped
- Orange (1 with peel, cut into wedges)
- White wine (1 c.)
- Whole peeled tomatoes (14.5 oz. can)

Instructions

1. Dry lamb and season with salt and pepper to taste. Warm oil inside a Dutch oven, and sear lamb on all sides, roughly 6 minutes each side. Move lamb to plate.
2. Place fennel, garlic, and onion in the pot and cook, until browning, roughly 8 minutes. Mix in wine and boil, deglazing the pan. Reduce heat and simmer until it has reduced 50%.
3. Toss in orange, bay leaves, tomatoes, broth, and cinnamon, plus the lamb. Simmer, then cover pot and transfer to oven set to 325F. braise for 1.5-2 hours. Remove lamb and place on clean plate.
4. Strain liquid left in pot, then return it to the pot to boil until thick, roughly 30 minutes.
5. Return lamb to pot to warm. Serve.

Mediterranean Cod

Ingredients

- Black olives (0.66 c., sliced)
- Cod (4 fillets, skinless)
- Fennel seeds (1 tsp)
- Lemon (1, sliced)
- Lemon (juice of ½ lemon)
- Olive oil (6 Tbsp.)
- Onion (1, sliced)
- Parsley (1 Tbsp., chopped)
- Salt and pepper to personal preference
- Tomatoes (0.66 c., diced)

Instructions

1. Warm olive oil at a moderate temperature, sautéing the onion with a pinch of salt until translucent, roughly 10 minutes.
2. Mix in tomato and olives, tossing in the juice as well. Allow it to simmer gently for roughly 5 minutes. Toss in fennel seeds and set aside.
3. Warm the rest of the oil in another pan and fry up the cod for 10 minutes, flipping halfway through until done.
4. Toss tomato sauce over heat to warm, then mix together the parsley, and serve atop the cod with a lemon slice.

Baked Feta with Olive Tapenade

Ingredients

- Baked pita or crusty bread to serve
- Feta cheese (6 oz.)
- Garlic (2 cloves)
- Green olives (0.33 c., sliced)
- Harissa paste (3 Tbsp.)
- Olive oil (3 Tbsp.)
- Parsley (3 Tbsp., fresh chopped)
- Roasted red peppers (16-oz. jar, drained)
- Salt (0.75 tsp.)
- Tomato paste (2 Tbsp.)
- Walnuts (0.5 c., halved)

Instructions

1. In a blender, combine your peppers, 0.25 c. walnuts, harissa and tomato paste, garlic, and 0.5 tsp of your salt until mostly consistent. It doesn't have to be perfect, but should be well combined.
2. Take half of mixture into baking dish that has been sprayed with cooking spray. Top with half of your feta, then spoon the rest of the red pepper sauce atop it.
3. Top with the last of the feta and bake until bubbly, roughly 25 minutes. Broil for the last 2.
4. While that bakes, make your tapenade. This requires you to combine your remaining ingredients together.
5. Remove mixture from oven and top with tapenade. Serve immediately with crusty bread or pita chips.

Chapter 5: 30-Minutes or Less Meals

Vegetarian Toss Together Mediterranean Pasta Salad

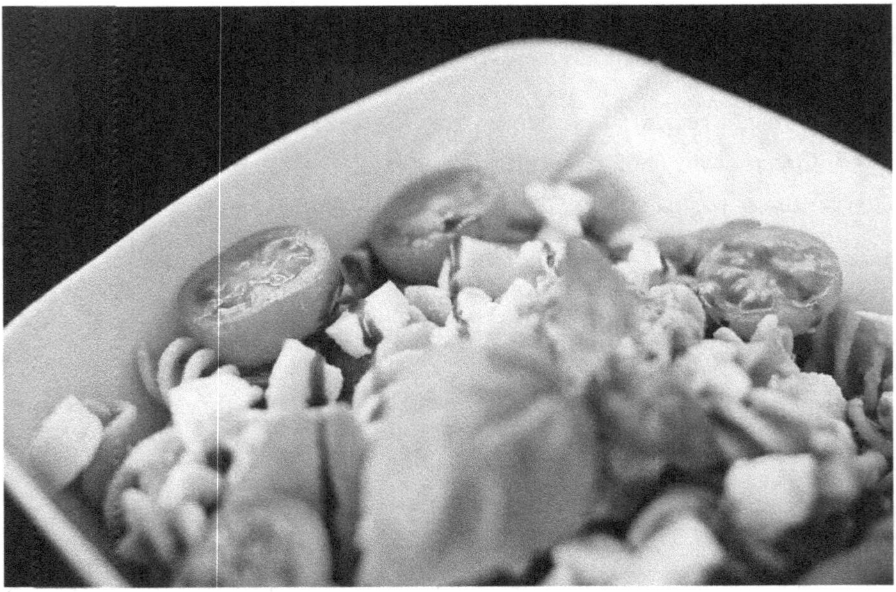

Ingredients

- Artichoke hearts (12 oz. jar, drained)
- Balsamic vinegar (2 Tbsp.)
- Kalamata olives (12-ounce jar, drained and chopped)
- Olive oil (2 Tbsp.)
- Pasta (8 oz., wheat)
- Salt to personal preference
- Sun-dried tomatoes in oil (1.5 oz. jar, drained)

Instructions

1. Prepare pasta according to packaging.
2. Mix together olives, tomatoes, and artichoke.
3. Drain pasta and add them to a bowl with artichoke mixture. Then, top with vinegar and olive oil, mix well, and serve warm.

Vegetarian Aglio e Olio and Broccoli

Ingredients

- Olive oil (3 Tbsp.)
- Cayenne peppers (3)
- Garlic (3 cloves, sliced)
- Broccoli (1 head, prepared in florets)
- Spaghetti (7 oz. whole wheat)
- Salt to taste

Instructions

1. Boil water and prepare spaghetti according to instructions until al dente. Drain and reserve.
2. In a pan, heat up 1 Tbsp. of your olive oil at a moderate temperature, then toss in the garlic and peppers, sautéing until fragrant. Remove garlic from heat and set aside.
3. Toss broccoli into pan and cook for 4 minutes. Then toss in spaghetti, garlic, and remaining oil. Cook for an additional minute or two, then serve.

Cilantro and Garlic Baked Salmon

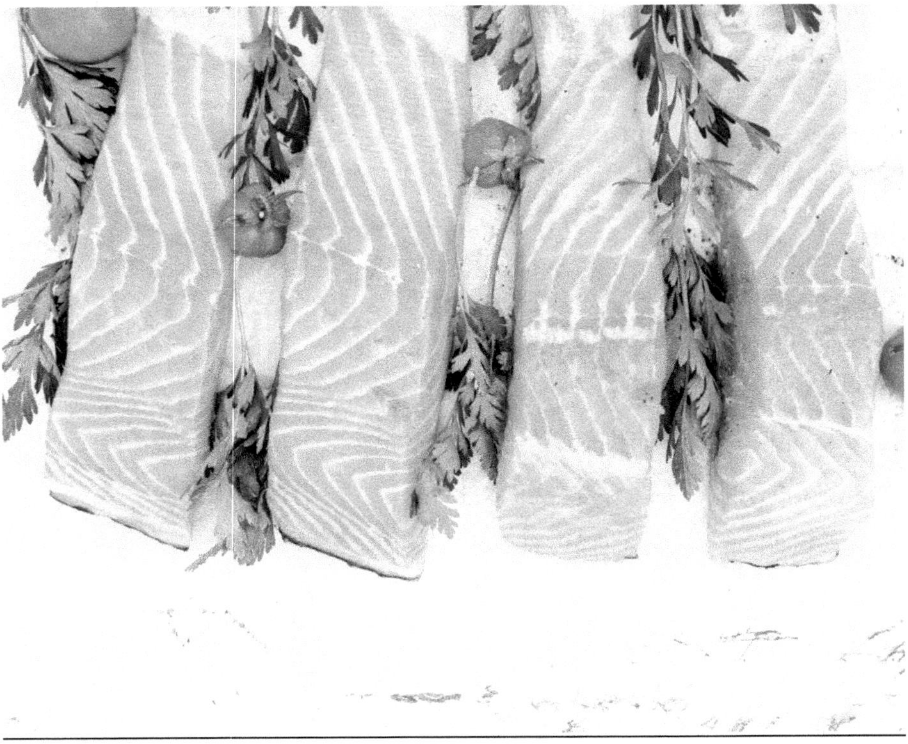

Ingredients

- Cilantro (stems trimmed)
- Garlic (4 cloves, chopped)
- Lime (0.5, cut into rounds)
- Lime juice (1 lime's worth)
- Olive oil (0.5 c.)
- Salmon fillet (2 pounds, skin removed)
- Salt to taste
- Tomato (cut into rounds)

Instructions

1. Allow salmon to come to room temp for 20 minutes while oven preheats to a temperature of 425 F.
2. While you wait, take a processor and combine garlic, cilantro, lime juice, and olive oil with a pinch of salt. Combine well.
3. Place fillet into baking pan that has been greased. Top with a light sprinkle of salt and pepper. Then spread cilantro sauce atop fillet, coating whole salmon. Top with tomato and lime.
4. Bake for 6 minutes per 0.5 inch of thickness (1-inch fillets take around 8-10 minutes). Let rest for 5-10 minutes out of the oven. Serve.

Harissa Pasta

Ingredients

- Pasta (2 cups)
- Red bell pepper (1)
- Red onion (1)
- Pine nuts (2 Tbsp.)
- Harissa paste (2 Tbsp.)

Instructions

1. Roast onions and peppers with olive oil at 400F for 20 minutes. Remove from oven and dice.
2. Prepare pasta to instructions on package. While pasta cooks, toast your pine nuts until browned in frying pan.
3. Drain pasta, leaving a touch of the water. Then, add in diced roasted veggies and harissa. Serve topped with pine nuts.

Chapter 6: 1-Hour-or-Less Meals

1 Hour Baked Cod

Ingredients

- Basil (0.5 tsp., dried)
- Bay leaf (1)
- Capers (1 small jar)
- Cod fillets (2 pounds)
- Fennel seeds (1 tsp., crushed)
- Garlic (1 clove, minced)
- Lemon juice (0.25 c., fresh)
- Olive oil (2 tsp)
- Onion (1, sliced)
- Orange juice (o.25 c., fresh)
- Orange peel (1 Tbsp.)
- Oregano (0.5 tsp., dried)
- Salt and pepper to personal preference
- White wine (1 c., dry)
- Whole tomatoes (16-oz. can, chopped and reserving juice)

Instructions

1. Warm oven to 375F.
2. In cast iron skillet, warm oil. Then, sauté your onion for 5 minutes. At this point, mix in all other ingredients but fish. Allow to simmer for 30 minutes.
3. Place fillets into skillet and top with most of the sauce. Allow to bake for 15 minutes until fish flakes.

Grilled Chicken Mediterranean Salad

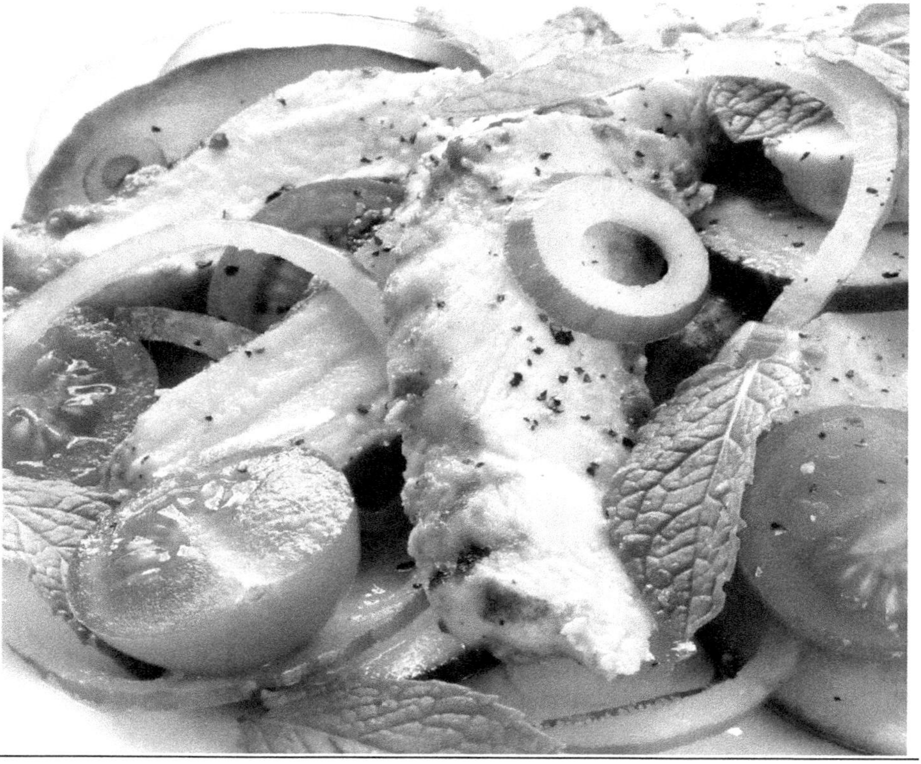

Ingredients

- Artichoke hearts (0.33 c., chopped)
- Balsamic vinegar (2 Tbsp.)
- Basil (1 tsp, dried)
- Chicken breasts (3, cut into bite-sized chunks)
- Cucumber (0.75 c., diced)
- Feta cheese (0.25 c.)
- Garlic (1 clove, minced)
- Greek yogurt (2 Tbsp.)
- Green onions (0.25 c., chopped)

- Kalamata olives (3 Tbsp., sliced)
- Kosher salt (0.5 tsp)
- Lemon juice (3 Tbsp + 1 tsp.)
- Olive oil (3 Tbsp. + 2 Tbsp.)
- Onion powder (0.5 tsp)
- Parsley (0.5 tsp)
- Pesto (4 tsp)
- Pinch of red pepper
- Roasted red pepper (6 Tbsp., sliced)
- Romaine (4 c., chopped)
- Shiitake mushrooms
- Spinach (4 c., chopped)
- Tomato (0.75 c., diced)
- White wine vinegar (4 tsp)

Instructions

1. Create your salad. Each plate should have a bed of romaine and spinach, topped with cucumber, tomato, artichoke, peppers, olives, and cheese.
2. Combine your tsp of lemon juice, wine vinegar, and pesto in a jar and shake to combine. Then, add in yogurt and 2 Tbsp. oil, mixing well until well-incorporated.
3. Prepare your chicken. Let it marinade in a mixture of 3 Tbsp. lemon juice, balsamic vinegar, remaining oil, and all seasonings for at least 30 minutes. Soak some wooden skewers in water during this time.
4. Make kebabs out of chicken and mushroom, alternating bite of chicken and bite of mushroom until chicken is gone. Grill for 10 to 15 minutes until done.
5. Drizzle salad with the vinaigrette, then place a kebab atop each. Serve.

Lemon Herb Chicken and Potatoes One Pot Meal

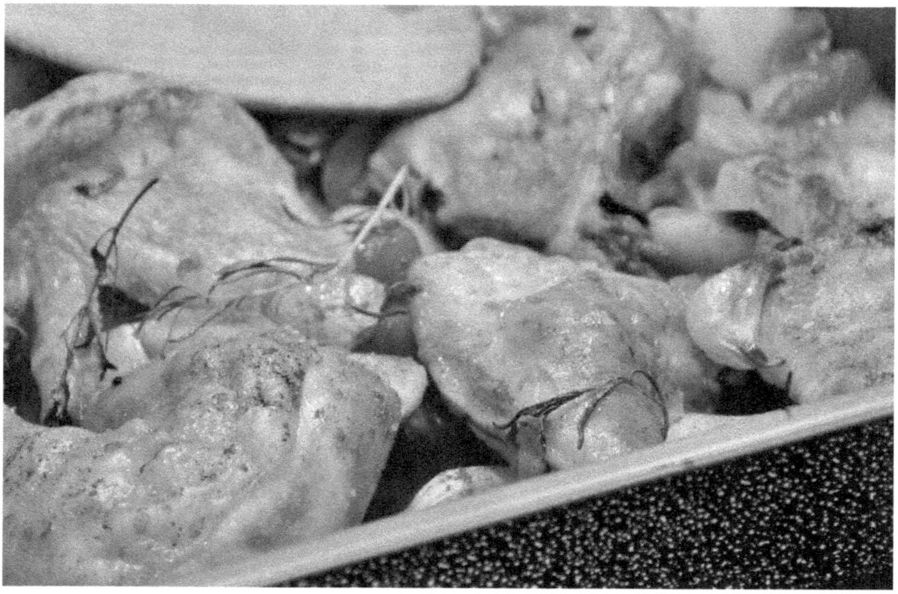

Ingredients

- Baby potatoes (8, halved)
- Basil (3 tsp, dried)
- Bell pepper (1, seeds removed and wedged)
- Chicken thighs (4, skin and bone on)
- Garlic (4 large cloves, crushed)
- Kalamata olives (4 Tbsp., pitted)
- Lemon juice (1 lemon's worth)
- Olive oil (3 Tbsp.)
- Oregano (2 tsp, dried)

- Parsley (2 tsp, dried)
- Red onion (wedged)
- Red wine vinegar (1 Tbsp.)
- Salt (2 tsp)
- Zucchini (1 large, sliced)
- Lemons for garnish

Instructions

1. Combine juice from lemon, 2 Tbsp. olive oil, vinegar, seasonings, and garlic into dish. Pour half to reserve for later, then place chicken in half. Let sit for 15 minutes (or overnight if you would like to prep the day before)
2. Warm oven to 430F. Sear chicken in cast iron skillet in remaining olive oil, about 4 minutes per side. Drain all but 1 Tbsp. of fat.
3. Place all veggies around the thighs. Top with remaining marinade and combine well to cover everything.
4. Cover pan and bake for 35 minutes until soft and chicken is to temperature. Then, broil for 5 minutes or until golden brown. Top with olives and lemon to serve.

Vegetarian Mediterranean Quiche

Ingredients

- Butter (2 Tbsp.)
- Cheddar cheese (1 c., shredded)
- Eggs (4 large)
- Feta (0.33 c.)
- Garlic (2 cloves, minced)
- Kalamata olives (0.25 c., sliced)
- Milk (1.25 c.)
- Onion (1, diced)
- Oregano (1 tsp, dried)
- Parsley (1 tsp, dried)
- Pie crust (1, prepared)
- Red pepper (1, diced)
- Salt and pepper to personal preference
- Spinach (2 c., fresh)
- Sun dried tomatoes (0.5 c.)

Instructions

1. Soak sun-dried tomatoes in boiling water for 5 minutes before draining and chopping.
2. Prepare a pie dish with a crust, fluting the edges.
3. In a skillet, melt your butter, then cook your garlic and onions in it until they become fragrant. Combine in the red peppers for another 3 minutes until softened. Then, toss in your spinach, olives, and seasoning. Cook until the spinach wilts, about 5 minutes. Take it off of the heat and toss

in your feta and tomatoes. Then, carefully place mixture into the crust, spreading it into a nice, even layer.

4. Mix milk, eggs, and half of cheddar cheese together. Pour it into the crust. Then, top with cheddar.
5. Bake for 50 minutes at 375 f. until crust is browned and egg is done.

Herbed Lamb and Veggies

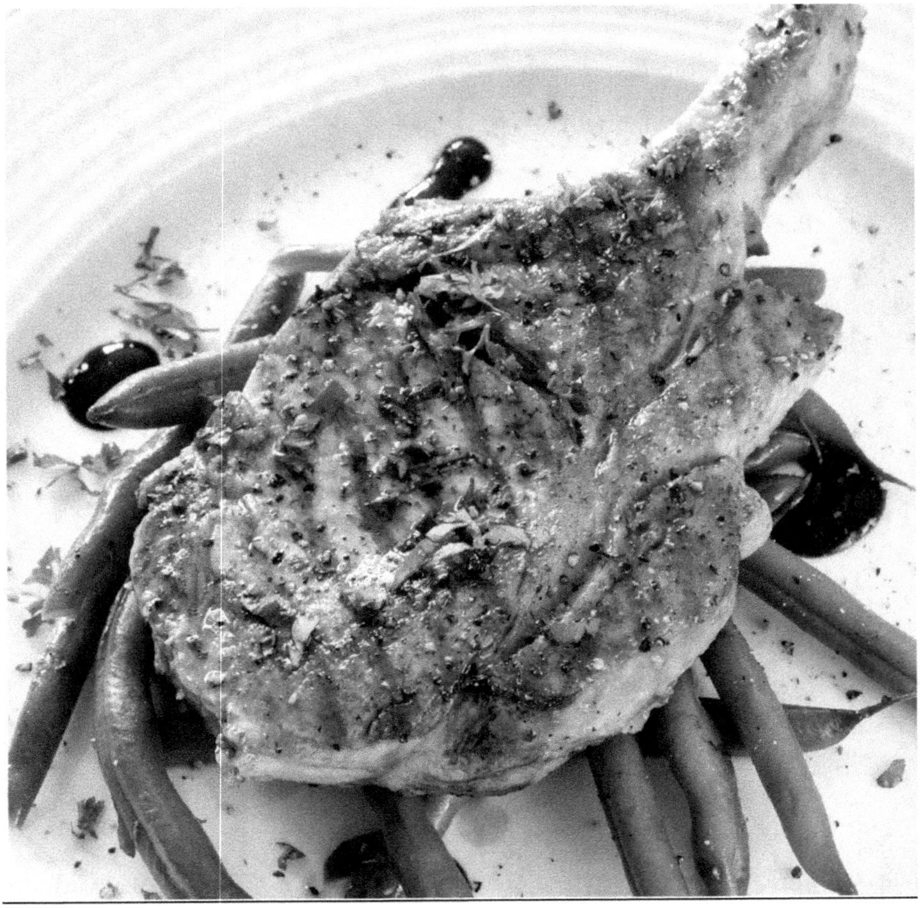

Ingredients

- Bell pepper (2, any color, seeds removed and cut into bite-sized chunks)
- Lamb cutlets (8 lean)
- Mint (2 Tbsp., fresh, chopped)
- Olive oil (1 Tbsp.)
- Red onion (1, wedged)
- Sweet potato (1 large, peeled, and chunked)
- Thyme (1 Tbsp., fresh, chopped)
- Zucchini (2, chunked)

Instructions

1. Assemble your veggies onto a baking sheet and coat with oil and black pepper. Bake at 400F for 25 minutes.
2. As veggies bake, trim fat from the lamb. Then, combine the herbs with a bit of freshly ground pepper. Coat the lamb in the seasoning.
3. Remove veggies, flip, and push to one side of pan. Then, arrange your cutlets onto the baking pan as well. Bake for 10 minutes, flip, then cook an additional 10 minutes. Combine well, then serve.

Chicken and Couscous Mediterranean Wraps

Ingredients

- Parsley (1 c., fresh and chopped)
- Olive oil (3 Tbsp.)

- Garlic (2 tsp, minced)
- Salt (pinch)
- Pepper (pinch)
- Chicken tenders (1 pound)
- Tomato (1, chopped)
- Cucumber (1, chopped)
- Spinach wraps (4 1o-inch)
- Water (0.5 c)
- Mint (0.5 c., fresh chopped)
- Lemon juice (0.25 c.)
- Couscous (0.33 c.)

Instructions

1. Cook couscous in boiling water according to directions on package.
2. Mix together your lemon juice, oil, garlic, salt and pepper, mint, and parsley.
3. Coat chicken in 1 Tbsp. of your mixture from previous step and top with a pinch of salt. Cook in skillet until completely cooked, usually just a few minutes per side.
4. Wait for chicken to cool, then chop into bites.
5. Pour the remainder of your parsley mixture into the couscous with cucumbers and tomato bits.
6. Place 0.75 c. of couscous mixture into a tortilla, then spread chicken atop it, rolling them up and serving.

Sheet Pan Shrimp

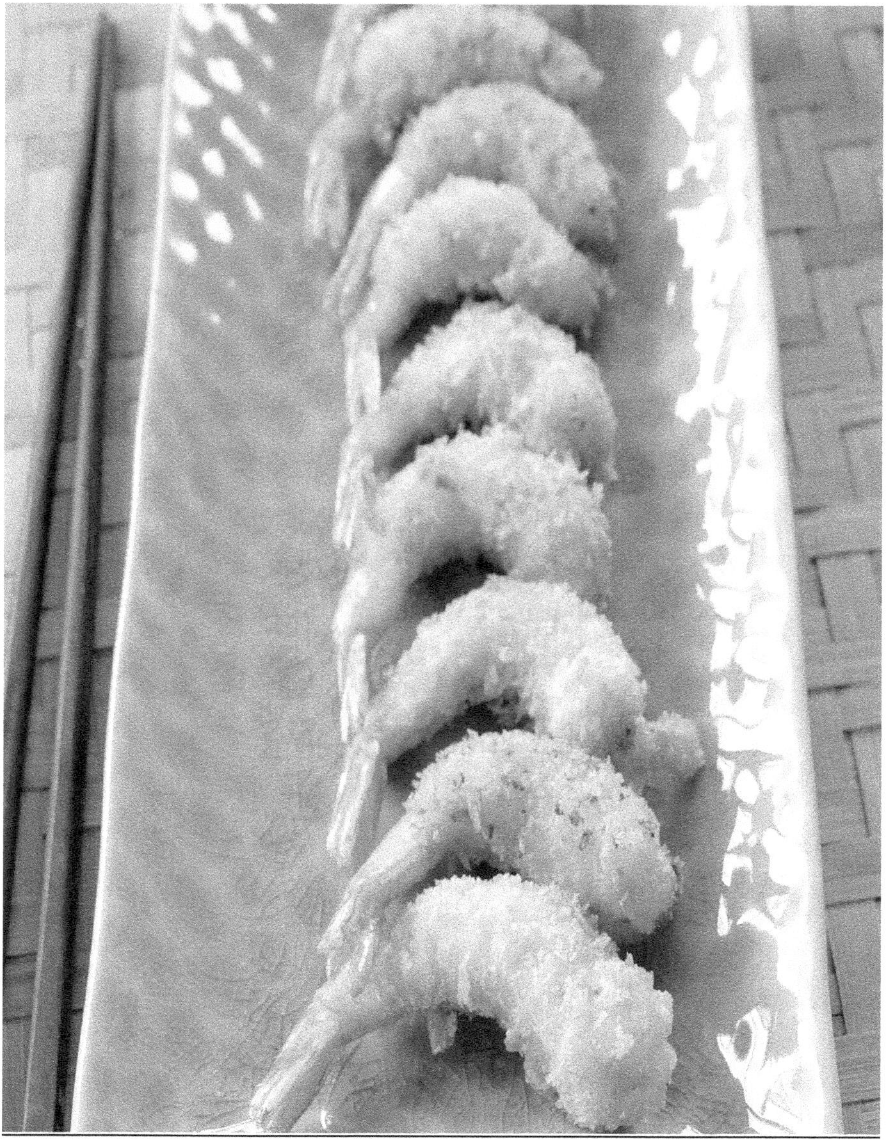

Ingredients

For shrimp

- Feta cheese (0.5 c.)
- Fingerling potatoes (2 c., halved)
- Green beans (6 oz., trimmed)
- Olive oil (3 Tbsp.)
- Pepper (1 tsp)
- Red onion (1 medium, sliced)
- Red pepper (1 medium, sliced)
- Salt (1 tsp)
- Shrimp (1 lb., deveined and peeled)

For Marinade

- Garlic (1 Tbsp., minced)
  Oregano (0.5 tsp)
- Greek yogurt (1 c.)
- Lemon juice (2 Tbsp.)
- Paprika (0.5 tsp)
- Parsley (2 Tbsp., chopped)

Instructions

1. Combine all marinade ingredients and set aside.
2. Take shrimp in a bowl with 0.5 c. of the marinade. Let them sit for 30 minutes.
3. During rest time, set up your baking sheet with foil or parchment, and prepare your veggies. Chop them up and toss onto baking sheet, drizzling them with the olive oil and giving them a quick sprinkle of salt and pepper. Bake for roughly 20 minutes at 400F, then remove from oven. Take out all green beans and set to the side.
4. Place shrimp in one layer across the pan and bake for an additional 10 minutes until shrimp is done. Serve with veggies and shrimp in bowls, topped with 2 Tbsp. feta and a spoonful of yogurt marinade.

Mediterranean Mahi Mahi

Ingredients

- Basil (6 leaves, freshly chopped)
- Capers (4 Tbsp.)
- Garlic (2 cloves, chopped)
- Italian seasoning (pinch)
- Kalamata olives (25, chopped)
- Lemon juice (1 tsp)
- Mahi mahi (1 pound)
- Olive oil (2 Tbsp.)
- Onion (o.5, chopped)
- Parmesan cheese (3 Tbsp.)
- Diced tomatoes (15 oz. can)
- White wine (0.25 c.)

Instructions

1. Warm olive oil in a pan and then cook onions until translucent. Toss in garlic and seasoning and stir to mix well. Then, add in your can of tomatoes, wine, olives, lemon, and roughly half of the chopped basil. Drop heat down and toss in parmesan cheese. Cook until bubbling.
2. Put fish into a baking pan, then top with the sauce. Bake for 20 minutes at 425 F until fish is to temperature.

Chapter 7: Slow Cooker Meals

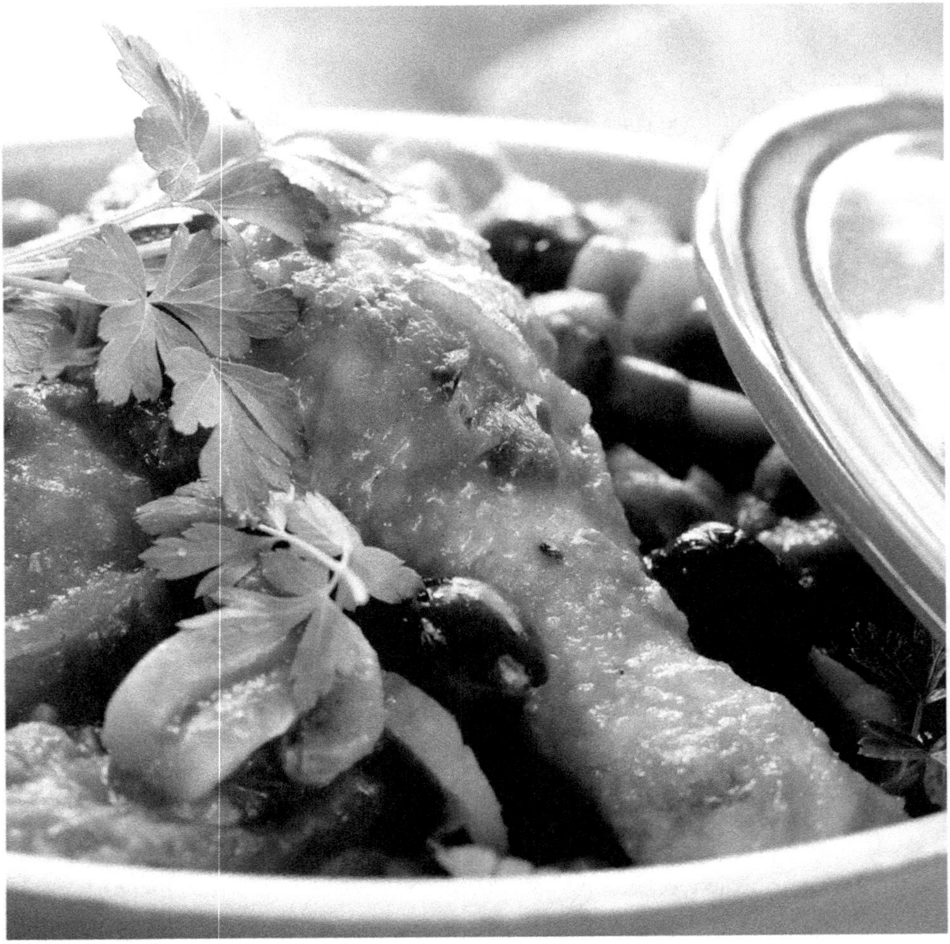

Slow Cooker Mediterranean Chicken

Ingredients

- Bay leaf (1)
- Capers (1 Tbsp.)
- Chicken broth (0.5 c.)

- Chicken thighs (2 pounds, bone and skin removed)
- Garlic (3 cloves, minced)
- Kalamata olives (1 c.)
- Olive oil (1 Tbsp.)
- Oregano (1 tsp)
- Roasted red pepper (1 c.)
- Rosemary (1 tsp, dried)
- Salt and pepper to taste
- Sweet onion (1, thinly sliced)
- Thyme (1 tsp, dried)
- Optional fresh lemon wedges to juice for serving

Instructions

1. Sauté the chicken in olive oil to brown on both sides, then remove it from the pan. Then, sauté the onions and garlic as well until beginning to soften, roughly 5 minutes.
2. Put chicken, onion, garlic, and all other ingredients into a slow cooker and leave it to cook for 4 hours on low. Season to taste.

Slow Cooker Vegetarian Mediterranean Stew

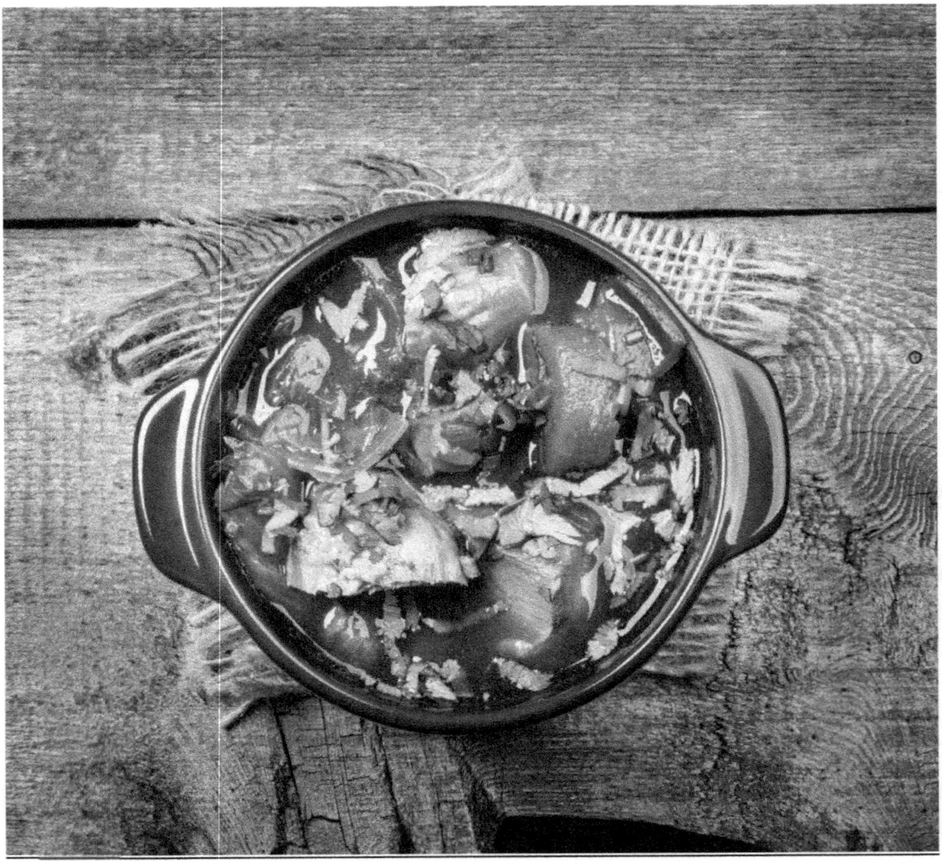

Ingredients

- Carrot (0.75 c., chopped)
- Chickpeas (15 oz. can)
- Crushed red pepper (0.5 tsp)
- Fire-roasted diced tomatoes (2 14-oz. cans)
- Garlic (4 cloves, minced)
- Ground pepper (0.25 tsp)
- Kale (8 c., chopped)

- Lemon juice (1 Tbsp.)
- Olive oil (3 Tbsp.)
- Onion (1, chopped)
- Oregano (1 tsp)
- Salt (0.75 tsp)
- Vegetable broth (3 c.)
- Basil leaves (garnish)
- Lemon wedges (garnish)

Instructions

1. Mix tomatoes, onion, carrot, broth, seasonings, and garlic into the slow cooker. Cook on low for 6 hours.
2. Take out 0.25 c. of the liquid in the slow cooker after 6 hours and transfer it to a bowl. Take out 2 Tbsp. of chickpeas and mash them with the liquid until nice and smooth.
3. Combine mash, kale, juice from lemon, and whole chickpeas. Cook for about 30 minutes, until kale is tender, then serve garnished with the basil leaves and lemon wedges.

Vegetarian Slow Cooker Quinoa

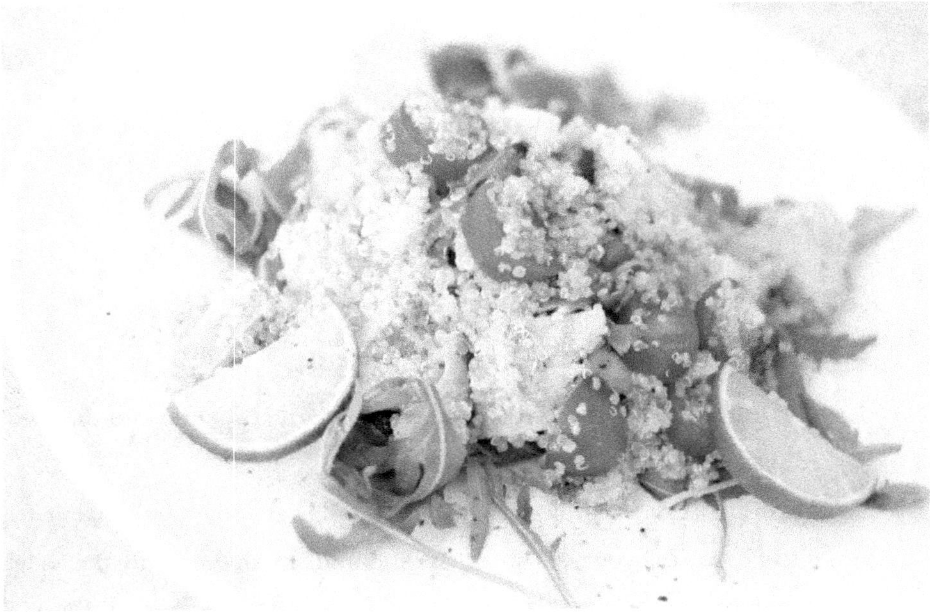

Ingredients

- Arugula (4 c.)
- Chickpeas (1 15.5 oz. can, rinsed and drained)
- Feta cheese (0.5 c)
- Garlic (2 cloves, minced)
- Kalamata olives (12, halved)
- Kosher salt (0.75 tsp)
- Lemon juice (2 tsp)
- Olive oil (2.25 Tbsp.)
- Oregano (2 Tbsp., fresh and coarsely chopped

- Quinoa (1.5 c., uncooked)
- Red onion (1 c., sliced)
- Roasted red pepper (0.5 c., drained and chopped)
- Vegetable stock (2.25 c.)

Instructions

1. Mix your broth with the onion, garlic, quinoa, chickpeas, and 1.5 tsp of olive oil. Sprinkle half of the salt atop it. Mix and cook on low until quinoa is done, roughly 3 or 4 hours.
2. Turn off the slow cooker and mix well. In a separate bowl, combine remaining olive oil, salt, and lemon juice together. Then, mix that into the slow cooker, along with the peppers.
3. Combine in the arugula and leave until the greens start to wilt. Serve, topping with feta, oregano, and olives.

Slow-Cooked Chicken and Chickpea Soup

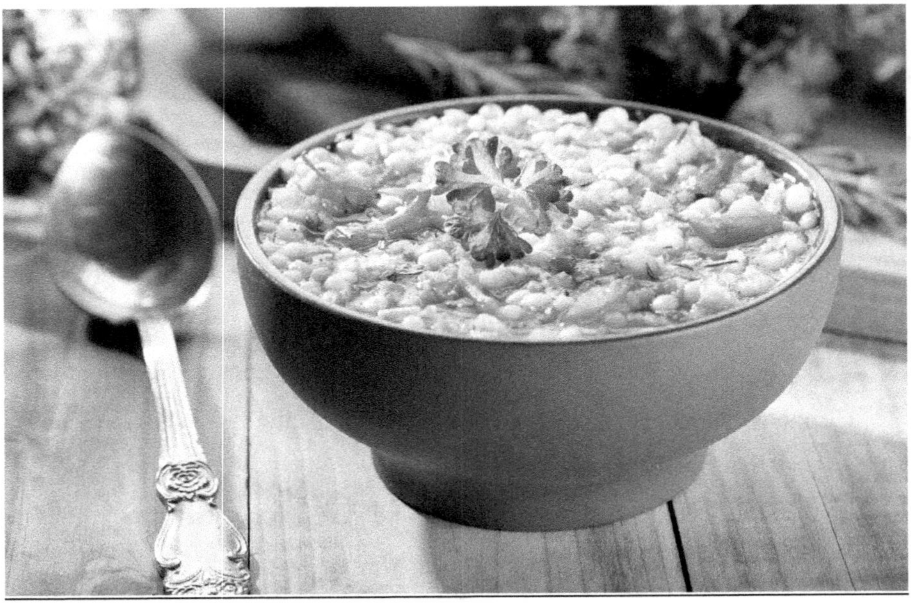

Ingredients

- Artichoke hearts (14 oz. can, drained and chopped)
- Bay leaf (1)
- Cayenne (0.25 tsp)
- Chicken thighs (2 lbs., skins removed)
- Cumin (4 tsp)
- Diced tomatoes (1 15-ounce can)
- Dried chickpeas (1.5 c., allow to soak overnight)
- Garlic cloves (4, chopped)
- Olives (o.25 c., halved)
- Paprika (4 tsp)
- Pepper (0.25 tsp)

- Salt (0.5 tsp)
- Tomato paste (2 Tbsp.)
- Water (4 c.)
- Yellow onion (chopped)
- Parsley or cilantro (garnish)

Instructions

1. Drain your soaked chickpeas and place them into your slow cooker (large preferred). Mix in the water, onions and garlic, tomatoes (undrained), tomato paste, and all seasonings. Combine well, then add in the chicken.
2. Leave it to cook for 8 hours at low, or 4 at high.
3. Remove the chicken and allow it to cool on a cutting board. At the same time, remove the bay leaf, then add in the artichoke and olives. Season with additional salt if necessary to taste. Chop up chicken, removing the bones, and then mix it back into the soup. Serve the soup with the parsley or cilantro garnishing the top.

Slow Cooked Brisket

Ingredients

- Beef broth (0.5 c.)
- Brisket (3 lbs.)
- Cold water (0.25 c.)
- Fennel bulbs (2, cored, trimmed, and cut into wedges)
- Flour
- Italian seasoning (3 tsp)
- Italian seasoning diced tomatoes (14.5 oz. can)
- Lemon peel (1 tsp., fine shreds)
- Olives (0.5 c.)
- Parsley for garnish
- Pepper (pinch)
- Salt (pinch)

Instructions

1. Trim meat, then season with 1 tsp Italian seasoning. Put it in slow cooker with the cut-up fennel on top.
2. Mix together the tomatoes, broth, peel, olives, salt and pepper, and the last of the Italian seasoning.
3. Cook at low for 10 hours, or high for 5.
4. Take meat out of the cooker and reserve all juice. Arrange meat with veggies on a serving platter.
5. Remove fat from top of the juices.
6. Take 2 c. of juices in saucepan. Mix together water and flour, then combine it into the juice. Cook until gravy forms.
7. Serve meat topped with gravy and garnish with parsley.

Vegan Bean Soup with Spinach

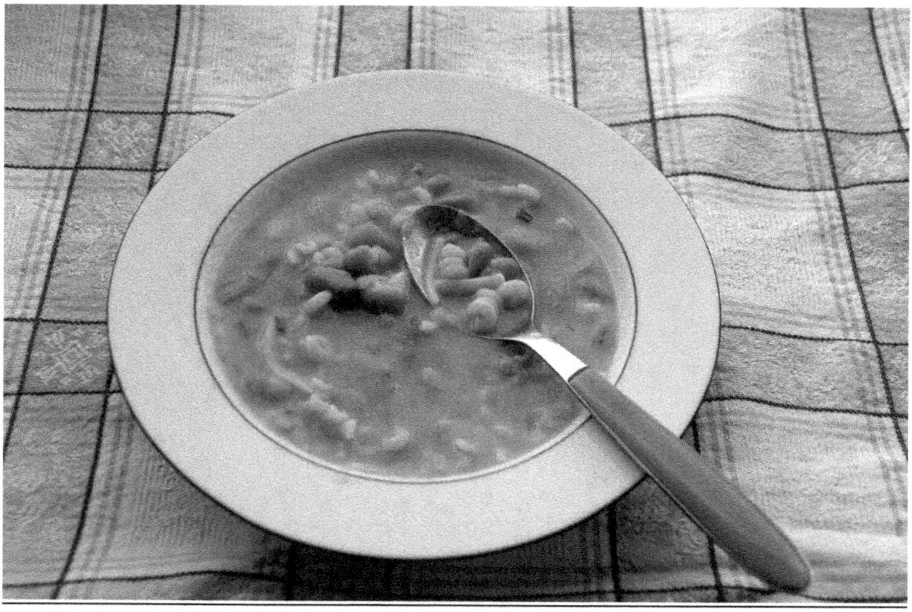

Ingredients

- Vegetable broth (3 14-oz. cans)
- Tomato puree (15 oz. can)
- Great Northern or White beans (15 oz. can)
- White rice (0.5 c)
- Onion (0.5 c., chopped)
- Garlic (2 cloves, minced)
- Basil (1 tsp., dried)
- Pinch of salt
- Pinch of pepper
- Kale or spinach (8 c., chopped)

Instructions

1. Mix everything but leafy greens together in your slow cooker. Cook for 5 or 7 hours on low, or 2.5 hours on high.
2. Toss in leafy greens. Wait for them to wilt and serve.

Moroccan Lentil Soup

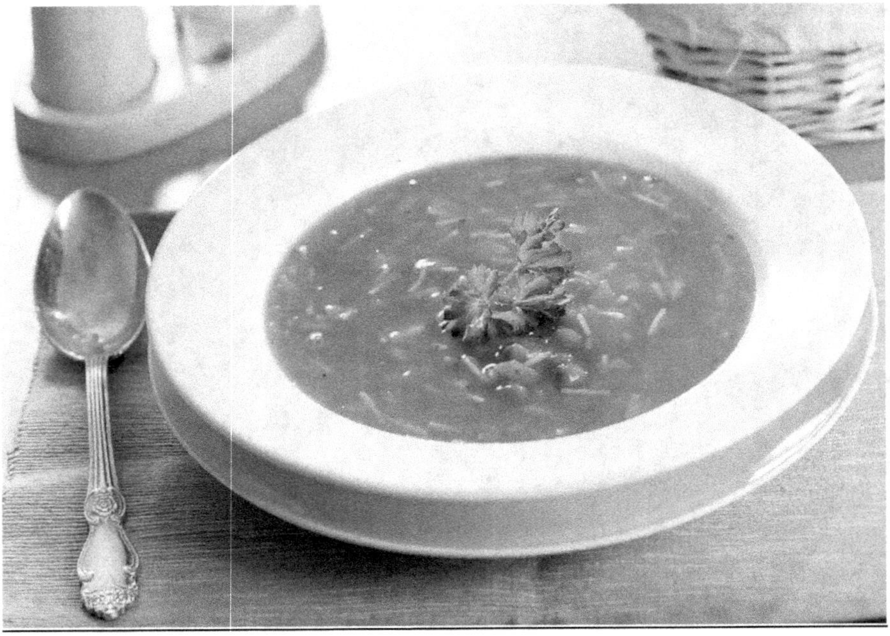

Ingredients

- Carrots (2 c., chopped)
- Cauliflower (3 c.)
- Cinnamon (0.25 tsp)
- Cumin (1 tsp)
- Diced tomato (28 oz.)
- Fresh cilantro (0.5 c.)
- Fresh spinach (4 c.)
- Garlic (4 cloves, minced)
- Ground coriander (1 tsp)
- Lemon juice (2 Tbsp.)
- Lentils (1.75 c.)

- Olive oil (2 tsp)
- Onion (2 c., chopped)
- Pepper (pinch)
- Tomato paste (2 Tbsp.)
- Turmeric (1 tsp)
- Vegetable broth (6 c.)
- Water (2 c.)

Instructions

1. Mix everything but spinach, cilantro, and lemon juice. Cook until lentils soften. This will be 4-5 hours if you use high heat, or 10 hours on low.
2. Mix spinach when just 30 minutes remains on cook time.
3. Just before serving, top with cilantro and lemon juice.

Chapter 8: Vegetarian and Vegan Meals

Vegetarian Greek Stuffed Mushrooms

Ingredients

- Cherry tomatoes (0.5 c., quartered)
- Feta cheese (0.33 c.)
- Garlic (1 clove, mixed)
- Ground pepper (0.5 tsp)
- Kalamata olives (2 Tbsp.)
- Olive oil (3 Tbsp.)
- Oregano (1 Tbsp., fresh and roughly chopped)
- Portobello mushrooms (4, cleaned with stems and gills taken out)
- Salt (0.25 tsp)
- Spinach (1 c., chopped)

Instructions

1. Begin by setting your oven. This recipe requires 400F for baking.
2. Mix together your salt and 0.25 tsp pepper, garlic, and 2 Tbsp. of oil, and use it to cover your mushrooms, inside and out.
3. Set the mushrooms onto your baking pan and allow it to cook for 10 minutes.
4. Mix together your remaining ingredients and combine well. Then, when the mushrooms are done, remove them from the oven and then fill them up with your filling.
5. Allow to cook for another 10 minutes.

Vegetarian Cheesy Artichoke and Spinach Stuffed Squash

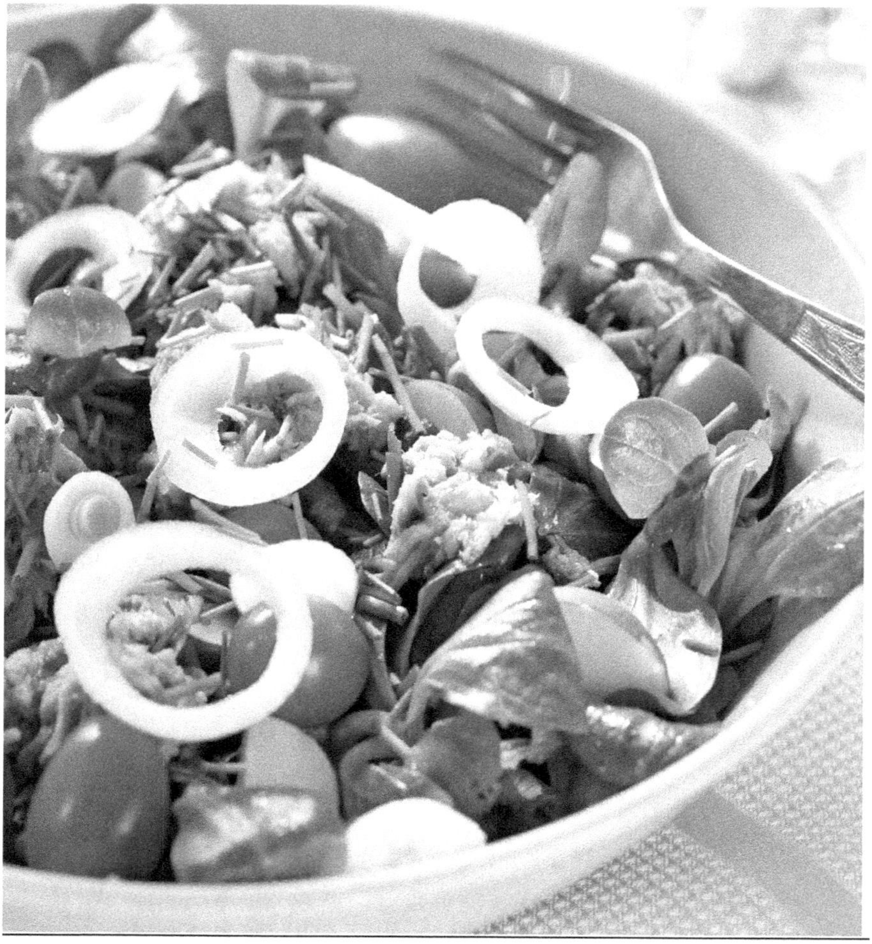

Ingredients

- Artichoke Hearts (10 oz., frozen—thawed and chopped up)
- Baby spinach (5 oz.)
- Cream cheese (4 oz., softened)
- Parmesan cheese (0.5 c.)
- Pepper (pinch to taste)
- Red pepper and basil (for garnish)

- Salt (pinch to taste)
- Spaghetti squash (1, cut in half and cleaned out of seeds)
- Water (3 Tbsp.)

Instructions

1. Microwave your squash, flat side down, with 2 Tbsp. of your water uncovered for 10-15 minutes.
2. Mix together your spinach and water into a skillet until they begin to wilt. Then drain and reserve for later.
3. Preheat your oven set to broil with the rack at the upper 1/3 point.
4. Remove flesh from squash with a fork, then place the shells onto a sheet for the oven. Then stir in your artichoke, cheeses, and a pinch of salt and pepper to the squash flesh. Combine thoroughly, then split it between the two shells. Broil for 3 minutes and top with red pepper and basil to taste.

Vegan Mediterranean Buddha Bowl

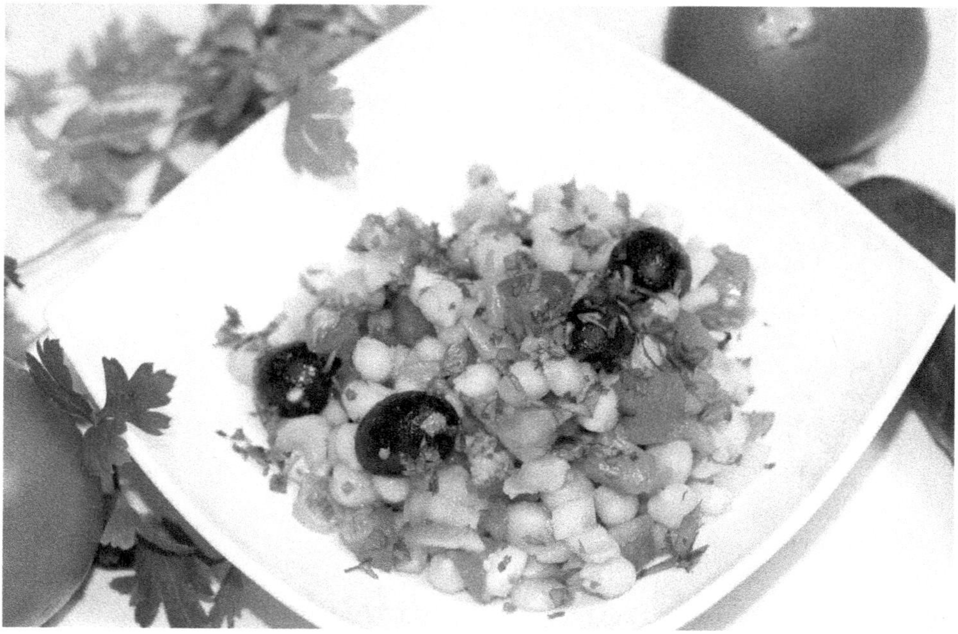

Ingredients

For the chickpeas

- Chickpeas (1 can, rinsed, drained, and skinned)
- Olive oil (1 tsp)
- Pinch of salt and pepper
- Dried basil (0.25 tsp)
- Garlic powder (0.25 tsp)

For the quinoa

- Quinoa (0.5 c.)
- Water (1 c.)

For the salad

- Bell pepper (1, color of choice, seeded, stemmed, and chopped to bite-sized bits)
- Cucumbers (2, peeled and chopped)
- Grape tomatoes (1 c., halved)
- Hummus (0.5 c.)
- Kalamata olives (0.5 c.)
- Lettuce (2 c. – can sub in field greens, spinach, kale, or any other leafy greens)

Instructions

1. Set your oven up to prepare for baking. It should be at 0400F. Then, mix the ingredients for the chickpeas together, coating them evenly with the seasoning.
2. Put chickpeas in single layer and put them onto the baking sheet. Roast for 30 minutes with an occasional mixing and rotation of the pan to allow them all to cook evenly. Allow them to cool.
3. Start preparing the quinoa and water in a microwave-safe bowl. Combine the water and quinoa and microwave, covered, for 4 minutes. Then stir and microwave for 2 minutes longer. Give it one final stir and leave it to rest in the microwave for another minute or two.
4. Begin assembling your salad. Begin with the greens at the bottom, then top with tomatoes, cucumbers, bell pepper, olives, chickpeas, and then quinoa. Finally, top with a dollop of hummus to serve.

Vegan Mediterranean Pasta

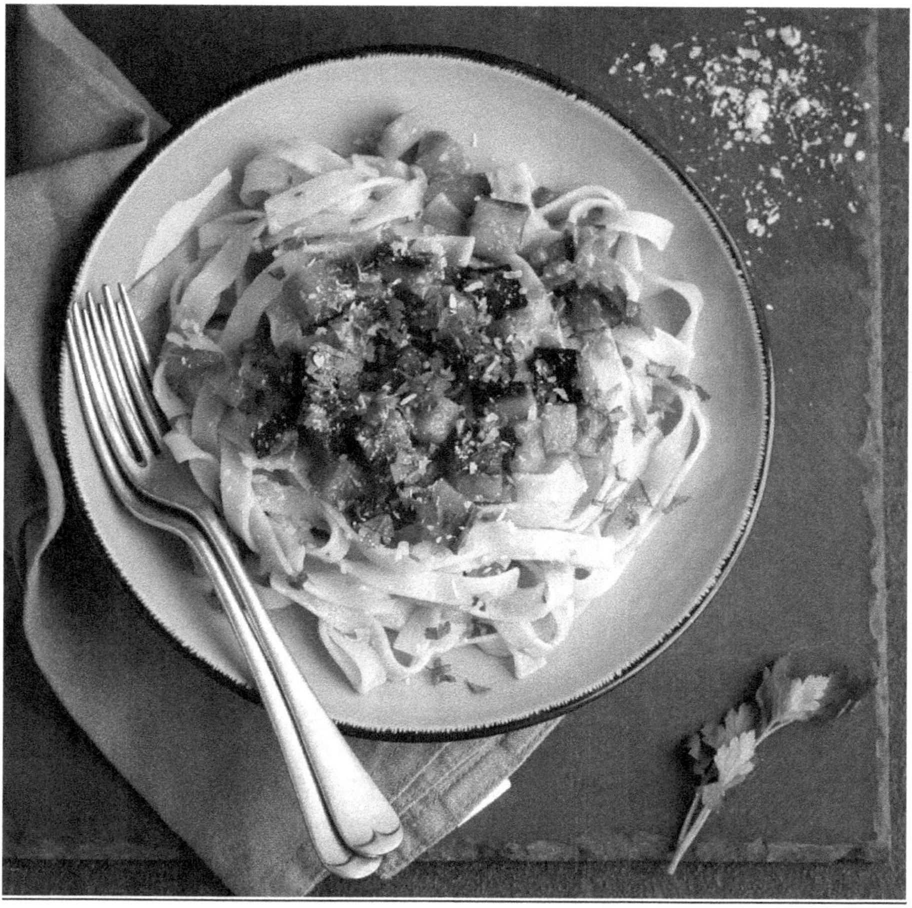

Ingredients

- Artichokes (0.5 c.)
- Basil leaves (0.25 c., torn)
- Garlic cloves (2-3 to taste, minced)
- Grape tomatoes (2 c., halved)
- Kalamata olives (10, pitted)
- Olive oil (1 Tbsp.)

- Pasta (8 oz.)
- Red pepper (o.25 tsp.)
- Salt and pepper to taste
- Spinach (4 c.)
- Tomato paste (4 Tbsp.)
- Vegetable broth (1 c.)

Instructions

1. Prepare your pasta based on the instructions provided. Keep 1 c. of the water for later use and then set the pasta aside.
2. While preparing your pasta, take the time to warm a large skillet with oil. Then, sauté your garlic and red pepper for 30 seconds or so. Combine in the tomato paste and cook for another minute. At that point, mix in your tomatoes, your seasoning, your artichokes and olives, and your broth. Let it cook until tomatoes start to break down.
3. Mix in the pasta to the tomato mixture. Let it cook another 2 minutes and add reserved pasta water if too dry.
4. Add in spinach and basil and cook until wilted.
5. Remove from heat and serve.

Vegetarian Zucchini Lasagna Rolls

Ingredients

- Basil (2 Tbsp., fresh)
- Egg (1, lightly beaten)
- Frozen spinach (10-ounce package, thawed and dried)
- Garlic (1 clove)
- Marinara sauce (0.75 c.)
- Olive oil (2 tsp)
- Parmesan cheese (3 Tbsp.)
- Pinch each of salt and pepper
- Ricotta (1.33 c.)
- Shredded mozzarella cheese (8 Tbsp.)
- Zucchini (2, trimmed)

Instructions

1. Prepare two baking sheets with cooking spray. Then set the oven to 425F.
2. Cut up your zucchini into strips lengthwise into 1/8 inch thick pieces. A mandolin will make this easier.
3. Prepare zucchini coated in oil with salt and pepper, then set up a flat layer across the bottom of the prepared pan.
4. Bake zucchini for 10 minutes until it begins to soften.
5. Mix together 2 Tbsp. mozzarella and 1 Tbsp. of parmesan. Then, in another bowl, combine egg, ricotta, spinach, garlic, and the remainder of the cheese. Toss in a pinch of salt and pepper and mix well.
6. Set up an 8-inch square casserole dish with 0.25 c. marinara spread across the bottom.
7. Take your zucchini that has been softened and begin to roll it. To do this, you will need to put 1 Tbsp. of ricotta mix at the bottom of your strip, then roll. Put the seam down in the marinara-covered bottom. Do this for all pieces of zucchini.
8. Cover the rolls with the remainder of your marinara sauce and top with the cheese mix.
9. Bake until bubbling, roughly 20 minutes. Rest for 5 minutes and top with basil.

Vegetarian Breakfast Sandwich

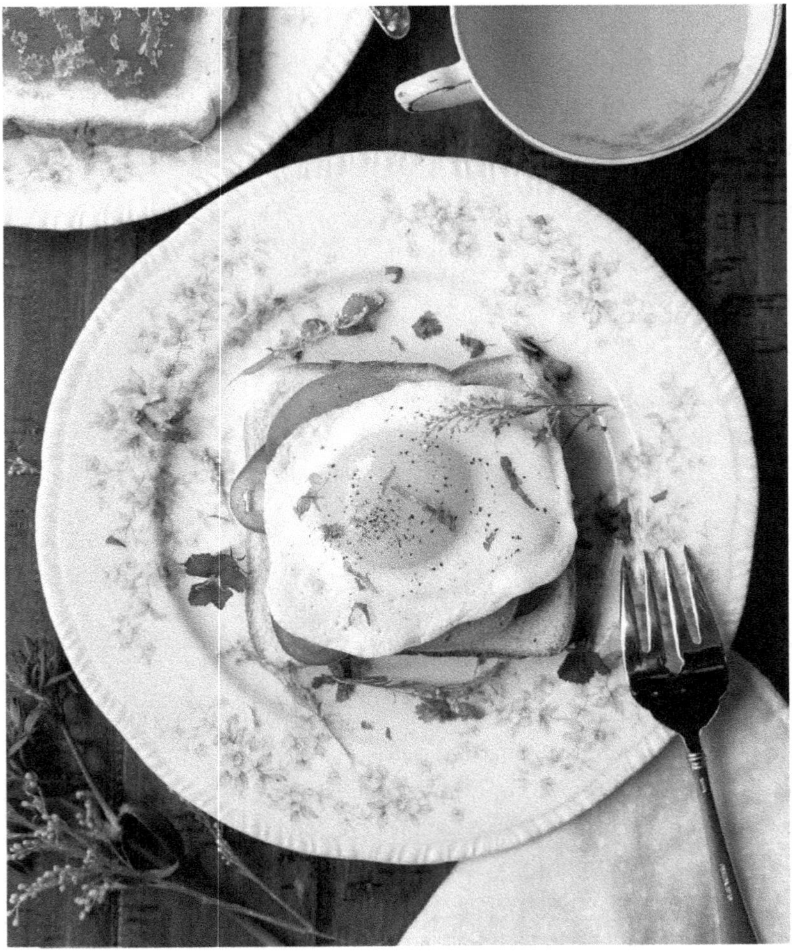

Ingredients

- Sandwich thins (2)
- Olive oil (2 Tbsp. + 1 tsp)
- Rosemary (1 Tbsp. fresh, or 0.5 tsp dried)

- Eggs (2)
- Spinach leaves (1 c.)
- Tomato (0.5, sliced thinly)
- Feta (2 Tbsp.)
- Pinch of salt and pepper

Instructions

1. Warm oven to 375F. Separate your sandwich thins and coat with olive oil. Bake for 5 minutes until beginning to crisp up.
2. Warm skillet with last tsp of olive oil. Break eggs into pan and cook until whites are set. Then, break the yolks and flip to finish cooking.
3. Put bottoms of the bread onto serving plates. Then, top with spinach, the tomato, one egg each, followed by the feta. Sprinkle with salt and pepper, then top with remaining bread.

Vegan Breakfast Toast

Ingredients

- Bread of choice (verify that it is vegan—2 slices)
- Spice blend of choice
- Arugula (handful)
- Tomato (1, cut into rounds)
- Chopped olives (1 Tbsp.)
- Cucumber (0.5, cut into rounds)
- Hummus (0.25 c.)

Instructions

1. Toast up your bread. Then spread the hummus across, season it, and top with all toppings split between the pieces.

Vegetarian Shakshouka

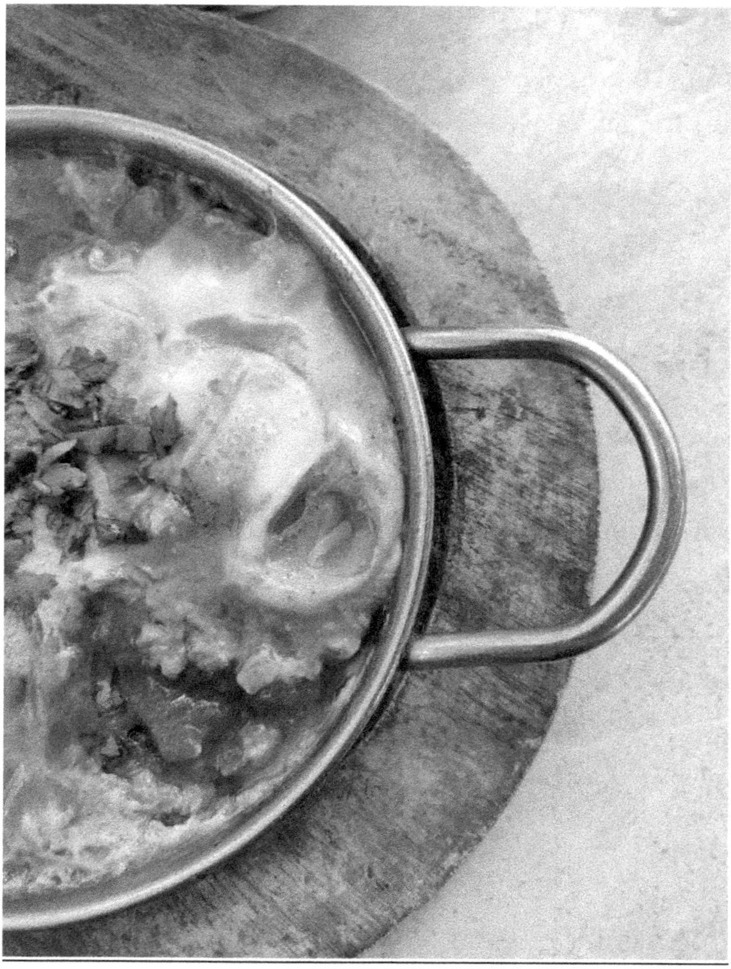

Ingredients

- Chopped parsley (1 Tbsp.)
- Diced Tomatoes (15 oz. can)
- Eggs (4)
- Garlic (2 cloves)

- Olive oil (2 Tbsp.)
- Onion (1—sliced)
- Red bell peppers (2, sliced thinly)
- Salt and pepper to taste
- Spicy harissa (1 tsp)
- Sugar (1 tsp)

Instructions

1. Warm oil in a cast iron pan. Sauté your peppers and onions until they have begun to soften, giving them a stir every now and then to prevent sticking. Add in the garlic for another minute.
2. Put in tomatoes, sugar, and harissa, leaving it to simmer for the next 7 minutes.
3. Season it to taste. Then, add in small indentations into the mixture in the pan, cracking an egg in each indentation that you make. Cover up the pot and allow it to cook until egg whites are done.
4. Cover with parsley and serve with bread.

www.ingramcontent.com/pod-product-compliance
Lightning Source LLC
LaVergne TN
LVHW012016060526
838201LV00061B/4325
* 9 7 8 9 8 1 4 9 5 0 7 6 3 *